CONFLICTED CARE

Conflicted Care

Doctors Navigating Patient Welfare,
Finances, and Legal Risk

HYEYOUNG OH NELSON

STANFORD UNIVERSITY PRESS
Stanford, California

STANFORD UNIVERSITY PRESS
Stanford, California

Library of Congress Cataloging-in-Publication Data

Names: Nelson, Hyeyoung Oh, author.
Title: Conflicted care : doctors navigating patient welfare, finances,
    and legal risk / Hyeyoung Oh Nelson.
Description: Stanford, California : Stanford University Press, 2022. |
    Includes bibliographical references and index.
Identifiers: LCCN 2022022353 (print) | LCCN 2022022354 (ebook) |
    ISBN 9781503611474 (cloth) | ISBN 9781503633476 (paperback) |
    ISBN 9781503633483 (epub)
Subjects: LCSH: Medical care—United States—Decision making—Case studies.
    | Clinical medicine—United States—Decision making—Case studies. |
    Physicians—United States—Psychology—Case studies. | Academic medical
    centers—United States—Case studies.
Classification: LCC R723.5 .N36 2022 (print) | LCC R723.5 (ebook) |
    DDC 362.10973—dc23/eng/20220628
LC record available at https://lccn.loc.gov/2022022353
LC ebook record available at https://lccn.loc.gov/2022022354

Cover design: George Kirkpatrick

Cover photo: iStock

Typeset by Newgen in Minion Pro 10/14.4

Contents

Acknowledgments

First and foremost, I would like to express my deepest gratitude to the physicians (both attendings and physicians-in-training) on the Internal Medicine Service at Pacific Medical Center for embracing me as I conducted this study. I am forever grateful that they shared a part of their lives with me, allowing me to be a part of the team during rounds. I am also thankful for the time they set aside to meet with me—during their lunch breaks, while on-call, and even during their days off. Without their interest in and active support for my research, this project would not have been possible. I am especially grateful to the director of residency training, who was particularly invested in this research. I would also like to thank the patients, family members, nurse practitioners, case managers, and other health care professionals at Pacific Medical Center who crossed paths with me during this study. I am so appreciative of the time they took to speak with me and allowing me a glimpse into their lives on the clinical wards.

This project has spanned my personal, academic, and professional career in many ways, so I have many individuals to thank. At the University of California, Los Angeles, I would like to thank Hannah Landecker, Edward T. Walker, Gabriel Rossman, and José Escarce for their support throughout my research. They enthusiastically met with me to discuss this project and read various drafts of my work, advancing it theoretically and analytically. I would also like to give special thanks to my advisor and mentor, Stefan Tim-mermans. Stefan read countless drafts, gave me vital critical and supportive feedback, helping me to complete this project. More broadly, his academic and social support and encouragement have been irreplaceable to me throughout my training and professional career.

Furthermore, thank you, Anthony Alvarez, Anthony Ocampo, Anup Sheth, Caroline Tietbohl, Lianna Hartmour, and Lorenzo Perillo for your support and friendship through graduate school and beyond. I especially owe a great debt to Sarah Morando Lakhani, Elena Shih, and Rennie Lee, who have been fixtures in my life from the first day I met each of them. They have been vital to my growth as a scholar—offering words of wisdom and encouragement throughout this process. And more importantly, they have given me moments of joy and adventure away from the computer and for that, I am forever grateful. I also am thankful to the UCLA sociology department's Health Working Group for their supportive feedback on this work.

I would also like to extend my gratitude to the sociology department at CUNY-Lehman College: Kofi Benefo, Chris Bonastia, Tom Conroy, Dana Fenton, Jennifer Laird, Madeline Moran, Shehzad Nadeem, Elin Waring, Esther Wilder, Devrim Yavuz, and Miriam Medina for your feedback and support both on this project and as I embarked on my first professorial posi-tion. I am especially indebted to Jen Collett, Susan Dumais, Susan Markens, and Naomi Spence for their advice, mentorship, and friendship over the years.

And, most recently, a thank you to the health and behavioral sciences department at the University of Colorado Denver. Thank you to my colleagues, jimi adams, Patrick Krueger, Meng Li, Ivan Ramirez, Ronica Rooks, David Tracer, Anne Marie Summers, Itzel Cervantes, and Sulastri Carr for embracing me these past few years. I am so grateful for your support of this project and of me as a scholar. Thank you to the HBS Doctoral students, especially to the members of the Qualitative Research Working Group and the Teaching Fel-lows. Conversations with you all (both academic and nonacademic) revitalize and energize me every single time. And a special thank you to Jen Boylan, Karen Lutfey Spencer, Jean Scandlyn, and Sara Yeatman for their friendship, mentorship, and support these past few years—I cannot fully express how much I appreciate it. I have grown immensely in my time at CU-Denver.

Furthermore, thank you to Stanford University Press and especially to Marcela Maxfield and Sunna Juhn for their ongoing support and commitment to this project. Marcela Maxfield regularly provided instrumental feedback, reading countless drafts and revisions, helping to make this a stronger book than it would have been without her guidance. Furthermore, thank you to the anonymous external reviewers who have all unequivocally helped me to improve this project theoretically and analytically. A version of Chapter 4 was published in the journal *Sociology of Health and Illness*, and portions of Chapter 5 were published in the *Journal of Health and Social Behavior*. Thank you to the journal editors and the external reviewers for their feedback on this research as well.

Special thanks to my long-time friends, Alicia DiValli, Camille Gray, Cristina Rivera, Douglas Hill, Michele Mustacchio, Nadjia Bailey, Nathalie Moise, Paulina Ortiz-Rubio, Shelley Han, Tatiana Ortiz-Rubio, and Toya Randolph for their friendship, support, and advice through the years. They have energized me, revitalized me, and supported me for decades. And thank you to newfound friends, Lauren Fine, Jess Wu, Rita Tarnate, Stephanie Shen, Simran Kaur, and Tsilat Petros, for your friendship and support this past year.

And lastly, I must express my gratitude and love to my family. Thank you to the Nelsons—Carl, Carmen, and Chris—who have showered me with love, support, and encouragement not only throughout the research and writing of this book, but more broadly throughout my life these past 13 years.

Thank you to the Ohs and Ohnerts—Ai Jung Oh, Mootak Oh, Soyoung Oh, Stephen Ahnert, Owen Ahnert, and Olivia Ahnert—who have been there with me every step of the way. My parents, Ai Jung and Mootak, are why I am who I am today, and I am forever grateful for their love and support of all of my passions and endeavors. Thank you to the Ohnerts—Soyoung, Stephen, Owen and Olivia—for your love and support through the ups and downs of my life. I would not be here without you all.

And, finally, thank you to Gabriel, Alessandra, and Paloma. Your cease-less support and unconditional love are what made this project possible. To Gabriel, special thanks for all of the conversations about this research, this book, and Sociology more broadly, and thank you for all of the drafts you read and the invaluable feedback you have provided to me throughout this process. But most importantly, Gabriel, Ale, and Palomita, thank you for the utter joy and love you bring to my life daily—you show me what is most important in life. This book is dedicated to the three of you.

CONFLICTED CARE

1 | DOCTORS' DILEMMAS

Prior to the autumn of 2010, Jordan, a 33-year-old man of African descent, had no previous medical history. In October, however, he began to experience headaches, weakness, fatigue, and fever. The symptoms became so severe that he admitted himself to a local hospital. What ensued were many hospital visits over a two-month period during which a full-body workup was completed. Infectious disease specialists and neurologists were brought on board after preliminary tests indicated lesions on the patient's brain. A myriad of blood panels, tests, and procedures were completed, yet the results remained inconclusive: infectious disease panels—including HIV—and two bone marrow biopsies came back negative. Even with numerous consultants caring for Jordan and a slew of tests and procedures ordered, the patient's condition remained unknown. He felt progressively worse over several months, and in February of 2011 brought himself to the Emergency Department at Pacific Medical Center (PMC). He was immediately admitted to the Internal Medicine Service after presenting with increased weakness, instability, and brain lesions.

Once admitted, the Internal Medicine (IM) team treated Jordan for his acute symptoms, and within a few days his frail grip, due to general weakness, and his limited movement, due to an inability to lift his leg, improved considerably—so much so that from a hospital administration standpoint he was fit to be discharged. Jordan's primary care team, however, was concerned about his pending discharge because his diagnosis remained inconclusive. They were suspicious that he may have lymphoma, but with all tests and additional medical workups still pending they could not be certain. Typically, this situation would not be worrisome, as most patients would already be scheduled for immediate follow-up care with all necessary physicians at PMC or another medical center. Unfortunately, Jordan was uninsured. His insurance status prohibited his return to the center and limited his other outpatient care options. With the uncertainty, and potential severity, of Jordan's medical status looming, his primary care team needed to figure out care options for him.

Outside the patient's room, Jordan's primary care team launched an intense conversation. They considered the best care options for Jordan and his potentially life-threatening condition. Christopher, the intern on the team, asked whether the patient, despite his insurance status, could simply remain in the hospital until all test results came in and a definitive diagnosis could be determined. Dr. Max, the attending physician, responded that this would be impossible because Jordan no longer needed any inpatient therapies (e.g., IV medications). He explained that if Jordan were to stay, he would be expected to pay out of pocket—leading to bankruptcy—or the hospital would have to foot the bill. Dr. Max reassured Christopher that this decision was not motivated by Jordan's financial status, explaining that even if the patient *was* insured, at this stage of recovery he would be released. Therefore, the primary dilemma the IM team had to address was not whether he could stay in the hospital but how he would receive follow-up care.

Jennifer, the team's second-year resident, and Christopher contemplated possible follow-up care options for Jordan. Dr. Max suggested that if the intern were to work at one of PMC's outpatient clinics that accepted under-resourced patients in the near future, he could take over treatment for the patient. Dr. Max explained that if Christopher were rotating at this outpatient clinic, the clinic could schedule an appointment with the intern directly and designate him as Jordan's primary care physician. Christopher unhappily responded that he was scheduled at other institutions and would not be rotating at the clinic for at least another month. The attending replied that one month was too long for Jordan to go without any follow-up care.

Dr. Max then asked Jennifer if she could act as the patient's primary care physician at the PMC-affiliated hospital she mainly worked at. Jennifer was hesitant, explaining that because of bureaucratic protocols, even as his PCP she could not simply schedule an appointment for Jordan. Rather, Jordan would need to go to the hospital's Urgent Care with a prescription that she had written for him and wait to be seen. Lauren, the team's case manager, reminded everyone that even with the prescription, the wait at Urgent Care typically lasted twenty-four hours. Unsurprisingly, many patients simply left without receiving medical attention. Jennifer confirmed that while this was the unfortunate reality of her institution's Urgent Care, *if* Jordan were to wait to be seen, from that point on it would be easier for him to make appointments with her. The attending dismissed this solution. He stated that this might be too arduous for the patient, resulting in his opting to forgo care, which would likely be fatal.

Lauren reminded them of a small free clinic in a neighboring area that used the same computer system as Pacific Medical Center. This did not facilitate access to records, but once the PMC records were obtained, the physicians could easily read and interpret the patient's medical notes. Dr. Max pondered this and eventually agreed that this would be the best option and that the patient should be directed to go there. Christopher voiced unhappiness with this decision—concerned that the clinic was not equipped to meet all of Jordan's health care needs—but eventually agreed with the proposed plan.

Extending beyond the typical five-to-ten–minute presentation and discussion of each patient during morning rounds, Jordan monopolized a large portion of the team's rounding time because of his uninsured status, tenuous follow-up care, and probable severity of his condition. Of particular note was Christopher's struggle to come to terms with the follow-up plan: he balked at a decision that he perceived as not in the best clinical interest of the patient.

This struggle to reconcile what Christopher wanted to offer Jordan as his physician and what actually could be done given the constraints of the patient's resources and of the US health care system is just one of many critical lessons that Internal Medicine physicians-in-training encounter on the hospital wards at Pacific Medical Center. These lessons, which are lacking in medical school education, expose trainees to the realities of practicing medicine in a system that is highly specialized, commodified, and bureaucratized.

In this book, I explore these lessons and their associated struggles, revealing a hidden curriculum of doctoring that manifests itself on the Internal Medicine Service of an elite academic medical center. While many of the lessons stem from the nature of current US health care (commodified care, specialized medicine, etc.), these lessons are further complicated by the dynamics in the medical profession itself as well as in elite academic medical centers, which juggle multiple conflicting institutional logics that inevitably shape the dilemmas that surface and the decisions that are made on the inpatient wards.

———————

"Do no harm" is the oath that health care professionals abide by as they enter a career in medicine. It represents the field's defining logic: the health logic. The health logic is the fundamental moral objective of the health care system, guiding courses of action for both professionals and institutions striving to preserve the health and well-being of all patients. Prestigious academic medical centers like Pacific Medical Center emerge as exemplars of this logic: extremely specialized, equipped with state-of-the-art facilities, and seeing highly complex patient populations. At such institutions, the nature of the patient population, as well as the facilities' capabilities, lead to the expectation that care will be exceedingly specialized, with opportunities to use different medical technologies and to provide therapeutic options typically unavailable in other settings. Upholding the health logic, however, is not always straightforward or easy, as seen with Jordan. No hospital or patient is immune to the financial and bureaucratic structuring of the US health care system or to the subsequent cost-cutting pressures that have grown since the latter half of the twentieth century. The field of medicine is entrenched with multiple, conflicting institutional logics that directly influence how health care professionals navigate care delivery[1] and consequently their ability to uphold medicine's health logic.

In Jordan's case, financial considerations and bureaucratic regulations— put simply, the market logic—became central to the medical team's formulation of his treatment plan. Jordan would suffer deeply if he had to pay out-of-pocket costs for care at PMC. Thus, although the decision to transfer him to an outside clinic may not have been the ideal choice from a prognostic perspective, it ultimately was the choice the physicians made to save Jordan from financial hardship. The salience of the market logic in the team's clinical decision-making is a critical reminder that hospitals are essentially businesses constrained by the financial structuring of the health care system; they must strive for efficiency and profit and cannot be expected to dole out free care to their patients. Furthermore, the legal logic, which may at first appear to be absent in Jordan's case, is an equally important institutional logic that shapes how IM physicians approach patient care on the wards. Concerns of litigation risk in health care and the shift toward defensive medicine make IM physicians at PMC acutely aware of their legal vulnerability. The legal recourse of patients is typically associated with sociodemographic character-istics such as higher socioeconomic status,[2] and Jordan's minimal resources undeniably shaped the team's ability to ignore any legal considerations when determining his care plan.

As the IM team pursued this particular case, the visible struggle of a first-year intern, who was trying to make sense of the limitations placed on the medical team, is juxtaposed against the senior resident and attending physician, who were both more accustomed to making concessions when providing care. These more experienced physicians explained to the intern that their decision-making actually served Jordan's best interest, despite not necessarily being given access to further care at Pacific Medical Center. While such considerations and compromises in care delivery are common, this experience can be especially unsettling for newly minted medical grad-uates like Christopher, whose primary focus has been on the mastery of necessary medical knowledge and skills. They are less familiar with how medical decision-making is inevitably shaped and constrained by a highly commodified and highly bureaucratized health care system.

How do physicians handle the conflicting demands of the clinical setting? This is not a new question in health care but one that numerous scholars have grappled with. Many have explored how medical professionals navigate patient care and medical decision making in a health care landscape ripe with conflicting demands and pressures. This complicated context routinely forces practitioners to come to terms with their inability to meet established professional and ethical standards,[3] often resulting in clinical and moral determinations that are situationally derived.[4] A common assumption may be that this difficult decision-making is most significant when physicians are faced with providing care for uninsured populations. Yet the reality is that financial, legal, and other institutional considerations are actually present when dealing with *all* patient groups, including the insured. For example, insurance coverage does not preclude denials of coverage as benefits vary extensively across different plans, leaving physicians with the difficult task of routinely having to negotiate health and market logics. One may argue that in such instances the health logic should unequivocally prevail and patients like Jordan should remain at Pacific Medical Center to receive the care they need. But what are the consequences for Jordan if he receives his treatments at PMC but is then left with an astronomical hospital bill that leaves him bankrupt?

The reality is that medical decisions are far more complex than simply following the mandate of "do no harm," especially as "harm" can take on multiple connotations ranging from physical harm due to inadequate care to emotional harm due to bankruptcy. As such, "health logic" can take on multiple meanings as physicians must consider numerous conflicting yet critical factors when making health care determinations because of the current health care system in the United States. Doctors always have to ask themselves, "How can I help this patient? What are the necessary steps? How can this patient pay for treatment in a reasonable way?" The patients in this book are ones whose situations do not allow doctors to use the most obvious (or most correct) answers to those questions, which leads one to ask: How do physicians make difficult choices as they encounter multiple logics in health care delivery? How do trainees learn to deal with conflicting logics, a dimension of care delivery that is notably absent in formal medical education?

This book looks at physicians' experiences as they encounter and learn to navigate contradictory institutional logics in the clinical setting. I argue that these logics give rise to a "hidden curriculum of doctoring" on the inpatient wards.[5] This hidden curriculum is a critical component of the socialization and professionalization of physicians, revealing the realities of practicing medicine in a highly commodified, bureaucratized, and specialized health care system, developed over the course of the twentieth century, transforming medicine and care. Early in the century, physicians represented the archetypal professional: they had solo practices, set fees for the services they provided, and maintained full jurisdiction over their work.[6] However, with the increased commodification and bureaucratization of care in the middle and late twentieth century, physicians, like many professionals, faced challenges to their autonomy and authority in the workplace,[7] becoming subject to interference from external parties because of economic and institutional transformations.[8]

Health care exchange was becoming less a direct fee-for-service transaction between patient and physician and more a complex marketplace encounter involving various third parties.[9] These third parties directly affected how physicians administered care by taking over tasks formerly under physician control,[10] determining costs of care, and placing limits on providers' treatment options.[11] The ensuing restructuring of care delivery also found physicians seeking employment in institutional settings—no longer able to simply hold solo practices.[12] Physicians were practicing medicine in increasingly bureaucratized and specialized institutions, where organizational goals of cost containment, efficiency, and patient-centered care were progressively factored into daily clinical decisions.[13]

As IM physicians continue their education on the inpatient wards during medical residency training, they quickly encounter hidden lessons that expose them to the new realities of care provision in an elite health care institution.

NEGOTIATING THE MULTIPLE INSTITUTIONAL LOGICS IN HEALTH CARE

Organizational theorists have long maintained that institutions are structured around a single or multiple institutional logics[14] derived from the broader societal context,[15] inevitably influencing the institution's actors. Some institutions—frequently referred to as hybrid—possess multiple logics that directly shape their identity, practices, and policies.[16] These logics drive day-to-day activities[17] and decision-making on the ground.[18] Hospitals are a prime example of hybrid organizations, often operating with numerous key institutional logics: health, market, and legal. Organizational scholars have theorized that the nature, and viability, of a hybrid organization is contingent on the compatibility of its various logics:[19] Do they directly conflict with what they are prescribing or do they align? Do they have equal weight in terms of the organization's primary objectives and goals?

When faced with multiple logics, the scholarship has generally found that either one prevails above all others or "intractable conflict"[20] emerges between them (deeply impinging on the organization's functioning), or that a "productive tension"[21] is reached where they coexist. Scholars have claimed that hospitals are especially prone to differentiation of multiple logics: different actors embrace distinct logics to meet primary objectives (doctors adhere to the health logic; the administration focuses on the market logic).[22] As one might expect, multiple institutional logics undeniably influence how health care practitioners handle patient care and make clinical decisions. Nonetheless, practitioners do exert some agency,[23] often drawing on experience and professional status[24] to cope with countervailing pressures.

Recently, however, microeconomic sociologists have argued that such explanations of actors negotiating multiple institutional logics and pressures are too simplistic to reveal the complex dynamics on the ground. The scholarship has long held an interest in exploring relationality in economic life,[25] with a particular focus on the complex relationship between morality and economic work.[26] Researchers have extensively examined how moral understandings impact market practices and transactions[27] and how such moral assessments, and the often emotional stakes associated with them, shape the ability of individuals to navigate competing economic goals.[28] This consequential decision-making, which is typically considerably varied, has garnered great interest particularly in clinical settings, where the decision-making process is highly complex and decisions are rarely if ever uniform, as health care actors grapple with conflicting professional and institutional demands. Recent scholarship has found that variation in decision-making can be largely attributed to actors' subjectivities when required to navigate morally ambiguous or charged situations.[29] In her study of discharge determinations in a post-acute care unit in New York City, Altomonte (2020) found that health care providers make vastly different determinations by capitalizing on the ambiguous nature of "independent aging." Independent aging has come to mean different, and sometimes contradictory, things for different patient cases, allowing for a wide range of discharge plans, which ultimately facilitate fast patient discharge from the institution. For instance, in some cases, independent aging translates to patients receiving additional assistance at home, and in others, it means the patient needs to be self-reliant. Altomonte furthers our understanding of moralism and economic activity by demonstrating how the concept of moral polysemy can "explain situational variation in moral economies... [as] flexible cultural concepts . . . become morally polysemous in specific contexts." Moral polysemy thus allows for "multiple normative expectations and economic considerations."[30] Through this process, individuals are seemingly able to adhere to a single broader goal or objective while also meeting other distinct yet conflicting goals.

I draw on moral polysemy to make sense of the dilemmas faced, and the decisions made, by IM physicians on the wards at Pacific Medical Center. I argue that the health logic, and the professional imperative to do no harm, is the overarching logic they use to handle the complicated care decisions they are faced with. As in Altomonte's work, however, almost immediately evident is what it means to adhere to the health logic *changes* across patients and situations. It may mean keeping a patient in the hospital at the patient's request, despite an opportunity for safe discharge and additional financial costs incurred by the hospital. It may mean discharging a patient after a life-threatening diagnosis because further care, while vitally needed, would risk leaving the patient in financial ruin. Or it may mean calling multiple consultants or running extensive tests on a patient even if deemed unnecessary by the primary care team. In all these scenarios, the clinical decision-making is rationalized in different ways and "good care" takes on multiple meanings: from ensuring a patient's satisfaction to protecting a patient from bankruptcy. What drives such variation is equally critical institutional logics that must be factored into the medical decision-making process. In this way, adhering to the health logic, and upholding "do no harm" becomes an ambiguous process that ultimately varies on a case-by-case basis, with physicians prioritizing different logics at different times.[31]

Decisions are further complicated by intraprofessional work dynamics in the clinical setting that obscure how logics are understood and privileged and how care decisions are made. The increased specialization of medicine, the emergence of new medical technologies, and the complex nature of chronic conditions associated with longer life spans have made collaborations among IM physicians and specialists an integral aspect of care delivery in the United

States[32] and abroad.[33] Furthermore, in the United States academic medical centers structure their care delivery around teams of physicians and trainees.[34] Teamwork is no stranger to health care, with scholarship showing that it is associated with improved patient outcomes,[35] greater patient satisfaction, and expedited care.[36] Successful interdisciplinary teamwork in health care settings requires shared responsibility and decision-making[37] and mutual respect.[38]

Predictably, however, teamwork is also associated with conflict. According to Abbott (1988), interprofessional jurisdictional conflicts are common when different professional actors vie for jurisdiction over a specific social arena (or in this context patient care). For instance, an overlap of skills among team members leads to disputes over shared tasks.[39] Disputes also surface as hierarchies develop,[40] undermining a team's ability to meet its goals as member divisions are reinforced, excluding particular individuals from decision-making and tasks.[41] At Pacific Medical Center and similar institutions, hierarchies are deeply embedded. The presence of trainees creates obvious hierarchies around training and experience within the IM team. In addition, the frequent use of consultations makes interspecialty care common on the clinical wards. Collaborative care and teamwork across specialties further elucidates professional hierarchies in medicine that extend beyond training, and highlight distinctions granted to different specialties and expertise. Intraprofessional dynamics on the clinical wards in academic medical centers like PMC inevitably shape dilemmas and disputes and how they are resolved by the IM team.

Intraprofessional work dynamics are particularly significant because of the highly specialized nature of medicine, with subgroups organized around different levels of medical expertise and technological sophistication.[42] The specialization of medicine increased in the post–World War II period in the United States. Three structural factors accelerated this process according to Starr (1982): (1) "no regulation of the size or distribution of the specialties"; (2) "hospitals [having] strong incentives to set up training programs for specialists"; and (3) "government subsidies, the high returns to specialty practice created by health insurance, and the lack of a corrective mechanism that would have reduced specialist incomes as their numbers increased . . . giving physicians strong . . . incentives."[43] One consequence has been that certain specialties are conferred greater status, prestige, and income than others,[44] often based on the perceived difficulty of the acquired knowledge.[45] These status differentials become particularly acute when physicians across different specialties must work together and share patients in settings like hospitals. Individuals higher placed in the hierarchy may exclude "nonprofessional issues or irrelevant professional issues from practice" in striving to maintain "professional purity,"[46] and this can negatively affect interdisciplinary teamwork on the clinical wards. In turn, IM physicians find themselves not only traversing highly central, yet contradictory, institutional logics but also struggling to navigate the intraprofessional work dynamics that exist on the Internal Medicine Service at Pacific Medical Center. Inevitably, numerous conflicting pressures and challenges collide, directly shaping how IM physicians navigate care delivery.

While all hospitals encounter conflicting health, market, and legal logics, hospitals themselves are not homogenous entities and are therefore shaped by various characteristics that influence how these logics develop in the clinical setting. In the United States, the overwhelming majority of hospitals are community based,[47] varying extensively in size and specialization. Some community hospitals are teaching hospitals. Some are highly specialized with more than five hundred beds, and others have six in total. Hospitals are also differentiated by how they are funded. Private hospitals are owned and funded by an individual or a group. Public hospitals are supported by local, state, and federal funds—for example, federal hospitals are overseen by the Department of Defense, the Department of Health and Human Services, and the Veterans Health Administration.[48] Unsurprisingly, conflicting institutional logics are largely shaped by the specific characteristics of the hospital itself.

Here I focus on one type of community hospital in the United States— highly specialized elite academic medical centers—and one population—US medical degree graduates, all of whom come from well-known American medical schools. I explore the institutional environment of inpatient wards and the experiences of physicians as they try to provide care on a daily basis. Academic medical centers are a critical fixture of health care in the United

States and have a unique mission equally important to providing medical care to the ailing: a commitment to educating the next generation of physicians. As such, they not only are made up of the health, market, and legal logics common to all health care institutions but are also associated with two equally critical institutional logics: training and research. Training in a clinical setting is vital to the development of future physicians: "Medical novices require the opportunity to practice skills under the guidance of experienced teaching physicians until they attain a high level of proficiency."[49] The training mission is integral to the identity of teaching hospitals, but it can generate incompatibility with the other institutional logics in health care institutions. For instance, medical training is associated with high costs, compromised quality of care, and increased legal liability.[50]

Research is another integral component of academic medical centers, with the University of Michigan being the first institution to combine medical education and research in the United States. Dating back to 1891, Dr. John Jacob Abel became one of the first physicians to devote his career to both medical education and research.[51] By the early twentieth century, Michigan had created a facility primarily intended for teaching and research. The tradition was solidified as other institutions followed suit. Clinical research has remained a primary goal of academic medical centers, even in the face of budgetary restrictions, with the Association of American Medical Colleges emphasizing the need for clinical research to inform best practices.[52] Although undoubtedly critical in any academic medical center, I do not focus on the research logic because in my observations it did not shape or define the dilemmas and interactions physicians regularly confronted on the Internal Medicine wards at Pacific Medical Center.

Although academic medical centers are unique, representing only a small subset of hospitals in the United States (approximately 5 percent), demographic characteristics fail to reveal the significant role these institutions play in our health care system. First and foremost, while there may be far fewer academic medical centers than other health care institutions across the country, they "conduct the vast majority of basic, clinical, and health services research"[53] and provide extensive care for the nation's ill. Statistics on care delivery support this claim: major teaching hospitals represent "71% of accredited level-one trauma centers[54] and 98% of the nation's 41 comprehensive cancer centers." They provide "69% of burn care unit . . . beds, 63% of pediatric intensive care unit beds, 19% of all alcohol unit beds, and 24% of all inpatient psychiatric beds."[55] They also provide "32% of all hospital charity care"[56] and are the sites for approximately "25% of all Medicaid hospitalizations."[57] Thus, academic medical centers are a critical site at which to explore the dynamics of health care delivery in the country given that they provide a great deal of care to patients nationwide and are typically the first to adopt new best practices in care provision. Accordingly, they can be considered "the heart of modern medical care,"[58] serving as a model of care provision.

Second, most physicians are trained in academic medical centers even if they then go on to provide care in other health care settings.[59] Thus, significant medical knowledge and perspectives on care are introduced in these institutions which frequently become the foundation on which trainees develop their professional identities and practices. Furthermore, non-teaching hospitals also encounter conflicting health, market, and legal logics, forcing physicians to constantly negotiate care decisions with these concerns in mind. The concerns may be different—for instance, learning to provide care in an underresourced hospital with few specialists and insufficient medical technologies—however, the decision-making process is similar: health care professionals must weigh the costs and benefits of care for both the patient and the hospital.

Accordingly, an argument can be made that the lessons learned during training deeply guide how physicians approach difficult care decisions in future clinical settings. Nonetheless, there are two critical caveats to be made. First, it is impossible to evaluate such medical training imprinting after students have graduated from their residency programs. Ultimately, it is hard to assess how much training continues to inform decision-making in work settings as a career progresses given that organizational contexts directly influence individual behaviors, actions, and experiences.[60]

Second, it is essential to remember that residency training is far from uniform in the United States, with distinctions across institutions, medical degrees (e.g., MD versus DO), and training (e.g., domestic versus international).[61] In her study of two US-based medical residency programs, Jenkins (2020) found that domestic and international graduate trainees encounter quite different, often stratified, residency experiences, with deep variation in what they are exposed to and what they learn. The implications of hierarchies and distinctions loom large as they feed into different career trajectories that place physicians in highly discrete clinical settings—for example, international medical graduates disproportionately work in underserved and remote areas. This book, which focuses on US medical graduates in an elite academic medical center, sheds light on the dilemmas and experiences of a specific population of American hospitals and physicians.

THE HIGH STAKES OF OUR CURRENT HEALTH CARE SYSTEM

Successful progression through the hidden curriculum of doctoring requires IM physicians to learn how to deal with multiple institutional logics. Given the constraints of the current health care system, this requires a multidimensional understanding of patient welfare. For instance, too often health care professionals underestimate the toll of financial insecurity on patients. When physicians fail to account for patients' financial situation, patients fail to comply with treatment protocols, forgoing necessary care because of lack of affordability. Or they receive treatment and then face financial destitution or a very legitimate fear of it, which can lead to poor health outcomes because of the physical and mental effects of stress. Physicians who learn how to operate in the health logic *and* the market logic can be vital to patients' health and well-being; by understanding the financial implications of care decisions, they strive to develop treatment protocols that are both physically and financially viable.

Hospitals are businesses, and without proper financial decision-making and recognition of legal liability for the services they offer, they can close,[62] leaving communities without access to health care services. In addition, recognizing how the health, market, and legal logics are interconnected can help health care professionals and organizations change approaches to care, helping to manage the nation's astronomical health care spending. When drawing comparisons with other Organization for Economic Co-operation and Development (OECD) nations,[63] the United States ranks first in health care spending as a percentage of the nation's GDP and per capita. In 2017 the United States spent on average $10,739 on a single person, compared with the OECD average of US$4,069,[64] exceeding Switzerland (US$8,009), Luxembourg (US$7,049), and Norway (US$6,351). While costs remain problematic, these numbers would be less startling if the US outperformed all other nations on basic health indicators such as mortality and health resources. However, this is not the case, with the US having an average life expectancy two years below the OECD average. Also, in 2012 the United States ranked twenty-eighth out of thirty-four nations for number of doctors and twenty-fifth out of thirty-four nations for number of hospital beds.[65] In 2017 the US ranked twenty-sixth for life expectancy and twenty-ninth for infant mortality out of thirty-five nations.

Unsurprisingly, the nation's health care expenditure has generated great criticism as spending increases continue—from $247 billion in 1980[66] to approximately $2.9 trillion in 2013 and $3.5 trillion in 2017—accounting most recently for 17.9 percent of the nation's GDP.[67] The 2008 *Dartmouth Atlas Report* intensified concerns about inpatient spending when it reported that the US health care system generated a great deal of medical waste that was preventable, much of it correlated with variations in treatments (e.g., use of consultants) and lengths of stay for the same condition across different US hospitals.[68] Unfortunately, patients in institutions that administered more care or held patients for longer periods—translating to more Medicare dollars spent—did not experience better health outcomes.[69] Accordingly, there are multiple ethical dilemmas at hand. One is that completely ignoring financial considerations in health care jeopardizes both patients' health and well-being and the ability to ensure a financially viable health care system for future generations.

Nonetheless, although it is necessary for health care professionals and organizations to understand the importance of multiple conflicting logics in health care, market or legal logics should not unequivocally prevail. Rather, it is important and appropriate for practitioners to be cognizant of conflicting logics when making determinations concerning patient health and well-being. Learning how to appropriately embrace these logics, however, comes with its own challenges because of various organizational and professional factors and constraints. This book reveals these tensions and this process as IM physicians are forced to tackle these logics on the PMC's inpatient wards.

REFORMING TRAINING AND CARE DELIVERY

The dilemmas and lessons that emerge from the hidden curriculum of doctoring demonstrate that the curriculum is not necessarily based on individual acumen but rather directly shaped by institutionalized culture, practices, and perspectives embedded in the training of physicians and in the structure of the hospital itself. Using rich ethnographic data, I uncover the challenges physicians face as they carefully negotiate conflicting pressures in care delivery. This data highlights the incredibly complicated, secondary context of decision-making in the inpatient setting, which illustrates why policy and program implementations to improve US health care delivery often fall short of their intended goals. And indeed, while a magic bullet policy or program that successfully addresses the ongoing dilemmas of our current health system is impossible, the data provides an opportunity to consider new directions for practice and policy that address some of the system's pitfalls, particularly in balancing patient health and well-being with the ongoing goals of efficacy, efficiency, and cost control.

The first recommendation targets the training and evaluation of novice physicians. Since I began fieldwork in 2010, it has become evident that interns begin their residency with little to no training in financial aspects of care delivery; medical education is focused on clinical knowledge. The few housestaff who are aware of broader financial issues, have acquired this knowledge by personally seeking out learning opportunities. This book demonstrates a need for medical students to begin to acquire a financial understanding of health care options and constraints—particularly for underresourced patients— early in their training, as their ability to overcome financial barriers in patient care has direct implications for patients' health outcomes. It is necessary not only to include financial components in the medical education curriculum but also to explicitly evaluate students on their ability to manage them.

Second, local, state, and federal resources must be provided to improve health infrastructure in communities in order to strengthen and cultivate partnerships between hospitals like Pacific Medical Center and various outpatient services and agencies that are vital for patients' ongoing health and well-being. Generating and strengthening local health care networks will have a great impact on patient welfare and inpatient costs. For example, transitions of care out of the hospital are a particularly vulnerable time for patients from a health standpoint—as many require ongoing follow-up care— and for hospitals from a financial one—as they are at greatest risk for financial consequences either with patients remaining in the hospital for too long or with patients returning immediately because of inadequate follow-up care. If hospitals can be more closely tied to local clinics and placement centers, this might help streamline transitions of care out of the hospital. Furthermore, a clear, established network can facilitate the training of physicians in affordable care options for underresourced patients to prevent delays of care and discharge that result when physicians are unable to secure follow-up care or place patients in facilities like nursing homes.

Third, national campaigns must be created to address the "more is better" approach to care in the United States. Task forces must engage in and evaluate research on care protocols across conditions and medical specialties. They must stringently evaluate how financial, legal, cultural, and bureaucratic approaches to medicine in the United States have shaped current best practices. Through this work, new programs must be developed at the national level to reduce unnecessary care. This will improve patients' overall care experiences while minimizing avoidable medical waste. Such programming will also help shift the current culture toward medicine and health away from heavy reliance on "doing more," which has largely emerged in response to cultural, legal, and financial pressures that have developed over time in the field of medicine.

───────────

In sum, this book explores what it means to practice medicine in the current era of commodification and bureaucratization, in which physicians must balance the often conflicting demands of cost-cutting initiatives, patient-centered care, fears of legal recourse, and bureaucratic practices and policies. I reveal how the clash of multiple institutional logics, made worse by intraprofessional work dynamics in patient care delivery, expose physicians to a hidden curriculum of doctoring that manifests on inpatient wards at one prestigious academic medical center. As physicians learn to adapt to this curriculum and its numerous lessons and dilemmas, there are direct implications for patient welfare and inpatient spending.

I draw from ethnographic and interview data collected over my twenty-six months on the IM wards at Pacific Medical Center from September 2010 to August 2013, with follow-up data collection conducted in the summer of 2015. Pacific Medical Center, located in the Western United States, is an academic medical center that often runs over its five hundred–plus capacity, with more patients than available beds. Internal Medicine, a general medicine service, cares for patients of all adult ages. I shadowed IM teams two to five days a week during their morning rounds and occasionally during afternoon interdisciplinary rounds. Many of the physicians preferred to be observed only during rounds because of their workloads. I also attended monthly IM hospitalist meetings for one year at either PMC or a PMC-affiliated hospital. A subset of these meetings was dedicated to improving the consultation process at the hospital. I attended meetings that addressed consultations with Endocrinology, Gastroenterology, Pulmonology, Cardiology, and Rheumatology. Lastly, I interviewed forty IM attending physicians and twenty-one IM trainees for a total of sixty-one semi-structured interviews. These interviews addressed physicians' experiences providing care on the wards, with a focus on general financial issues that pervade care delivery, working with colleagues, and hospital disposition.

Chapter 2 introduces the Pacific Medical Center and offers a brief overview of teaching hospitals in the United States. It explores in detail the conflicting institutional logics at PMC, examining how they create a working environment that gives way to a hidden curriculum of doctoring. Particular focus is placed on the conflicting objectives, pressures, and dilemmas that IM physicians must learn to deal with while providing care on the wards.

Chapters 3 through 5 explore how the hidden curriculum develops through a specific aspect of care delivery: respectively medical notation, consultations, and discharge. Chapter 3 reveals how IM physicians encounter the multiple institutional logics at Pacific Medical Center via notation. The medical record is shown to be where physicians are made acutely aware of the contradictory nature of medicine's health, market, and legal logics. Physicians realize that proper medical notation is vital to preserving the health logic, ensuring patient health and well-being. Yet the medical record also exposes physicians to third-party payers in health care delivery and to their own vulnerability to litigation risk. This reminds physicians that proper medical notation is not simply proper clinical documentation but a much more careful crafting of information and clinical decision-making that accounts for the often contradictory pressures of multiple institutional logics.

Chapter 4 explores how multiple institutional logics drive the heavy reliance on interspecialty care on the IM wards. IM physicians are pressured to share their patients with consultants in the name of patient health and well-being. Although the assumption is that consultations benefit the hospital's health logic (improving care and patient outcomes), interspecialty care is largely driven by the hospital's market and legal logics, frequently compromising the objectives of the health logic, which is often even further compromised by work dynamics created by PMC's organizational culture and the medical profession's intraprofessional status hierarchies. This leads to unintended consequences for patient, physician, and hospital—jeopardizing all of the hospital's institutional logics. Portions of this chapter have been published in the *Sociology of Health and Illness*.

Chapter 5 explores the multifaceted, and highly charged, nature of hospital discharge management at Pacific Medical Center. Discharge decisions are never simple determinations of patient departure dates but rather careful negotiations between patients, families, physicians, insurers, and other relevant third parties. Discharge is arguably the aspect of care delivery where the contradictory objectives of the health, market, legal, and training logics are most acutely experienced by IM physicians. As the medical team strives to meet the objectives of one logic through discharge management, its decisions frequently compromise the objectives of another one (e.g., extending a patient's stay at the financial expense of the hospital). Thus, IM physicians must learn to carefully weigh and balance the contradictory logics when making discharge decisions, resulting in determinations that are rarely uniform and instead are situational. Portions of this chapter have been published in the *Journal of Health and Social Behavior*.

Chapter 6 concludes the book with an examination of how the multiple central yet contradictory institutional logics lead to unintended financial consequences for the hospital and the broader health care system. It reveals how the hidden curriculum of doctoring on the inpatient wards—and its associated learning curve—generate avoidable costs for both patient and hospital. I reflect on the conditions that promote this hidden curriculum of doctoring and the possibility for change to effectively address some of the shortcomings of health care in the United States. I conclude with some practice and policy recommendations for practitioners, policymakers, and institutions.

Appendix I provides a discussion of my methodology and my personal ethnographic experiences in the field. Appendix II offers a glossary of terms.

2 | CONFLICTING LOGICS

Pacific Medical Center, designated a level-1 trauma center, stands out prominently in the neighborhood as a bastion of medicine, science, technology, and education. Its modern, clean-cut exteriors and glittering glass windows remind all who pass by of the extraordinary capabilities of medicine to preserve health and well-being. The multiple glass doors open to an immaculate and bustling, lobby. Volunteers and hospital staff greet and direct visitors unsure of where to go. Seating areas are filled with individuals—some dressed in professional attire waiting for meetings and appointments; others laden with flowers, snacks, and balloons for their loved ones who are staying at the hospital. Health care professionals briskly walk in teams immersed in conversation, some enter the cafeteria for a quick break, and others travel from the Emergency Department and Observation units to the elevators.

Similar to the lobby, the hallway on the third floor of the center, where Internal Medicine is primarily housed, is always busy. Patients are out and about completing their morning exercise, gingerly walking the halls in socks, with an aide or a family member. Visitors roam the halls. Dining Services staff pick up empty meal trays and janitors empty waste baskets. A jolly tune reverberates through the halls signaling that someone needs assistance. Nurses work at computer stations or administer therapies in patient rooms. The low hum of numerous conversations can be heard throughout. Several

Internal Medicine (IM) teams are scattered in the hallway, discussing their patients, crossing paths as they proceed through their morning rounds.

The pristine building, the crowded lobby, and the large medical teams reflect the nature of the institution: Pacific Medical Center (PMC) is an elite hospital with state-of-the-art medical technologies and services. Unsurprisingly, people travel across the world to receive care here. Furthermore, it is a top training center for physicians; medical students, interns, and residents are fixtures, readily visible throughout.

As a prestigious academic medical center, PMC has unique objectives and challenges because of its multidimensional identity as a caregiving institution, a business, and a training center. Each dimension operates with clearly defined prerogatives and goals. Unlike organizations that have one primary institutional logic that organizes their overarching objectives and responsibilities, PMC, like others of its kind, comprises health, market, legal, research, and training logics.[1] These logics, while central to the organization's varied goals, create contradictory dilemmas for those who work at the center. For instance, what is best for the patient from a health perspective may not be what is financially feasible for the hospital from a market perspective, or it may leave the hospital vulnerable to malpractice litigation. Furthermore, institutions like Pacific Medical Center have the added responsibility of training future physicians. The training logic further complicates considerations that must be factored into care decision-making. This complex working environment drives the hidden curriculum of doctoring on the clinical wards where doctors must learn to reconcile the varied logics as they work to meet the care needs of their patients. In the following three chapters, I focus on the lessons learned through three key components of care delivery: medical notation, consultations, and discharge management.

While the doctoring curriculum is vital to the professionalization of trainees, it is not necessarily experienced uniformly by team members. Rather, its lessons and dilemmas are differentiated based on the level of training and practice on the IM team. As I observed in my fieldwork, on each team there were one to two medical students, two interns, one resident, and one attending physician. Medical students were in their third and fourth year of medical school, rotating on the clinical wards to determine their residency preferences. The interns were in their first year of residency; the residents, in their second or third year. Collectively, the trainees are often referred to as the housestaff.[2] The IM residency at Pacific Medical Center, like all IM training programs in the United States, is three years. Internal Medicine is "the study and practice of health promotion, disease prevention, diagnosis, care, and treatment of men and women from adolescence to old age, during health and all stages of illness."[3] As a generalist service, its interns and residents are required to learn not only specific procedures and therapies but also how to make a broad range of medical decisions (from differential diagnosis to possible prognosis). While the team works together supervised by the attending, medical students primarily report to interns; interns, to the resident; and the resident, to the attending.

Each team covers twenty patients on the IM wards, with ten assigned to each intern. Residents oversee care for all patients. Housestaff are therefore responsible for the bulk of the day-to-day medical work as part of their continuing medical education. As they carry out their daily tasks, trainees quickly encounter dilemmas that stem from the multiple conflicting logics at Pacific Medical Center. As IM physicians work their way through this curriculum, critical socialization and professionalization lessons are learned. Before I look at how the curriculum of doctoring reveals itself through the different facets of care delivery in subsequent chapters, in this one I provide a foundational overview of the institutional logics that are particularly significant in the clinical setting. First, however, is a brief historical discussion of hospitals in the United States and then a discussion of the institutional logics and how they directly shape care delivery on the IM wards at Pacific Medical Center.

AMERICAN HOSPITALS: A BRIEF HISTORY

The first general hospital in the United States opened in 1752 in Pennsylvania. Shortly thereafter, in 1771, New York Hospital was chartered and eventually opened in 1791. In 1821, Massachusetts General Hospital opened its doors. During this preindustrial period, hospitals were primarily religious and charitable institutions that offered care to the poor. Other than federally run marine hospitals,[4] these hospitals were public institutions, often derived from almshouses,[5] that served the homeless, the poor, and the mentally ill. The early nineteenth century was when hospitals operated primarily according to the health logic: the commitment of care dictated care delivery. The market logic, in contrast, played a rather minimal role at this time; institutions ran on voluntary donations—which required proper management of course— but financial considerations were not a central feature of the hospital itself.

Over the course of the nineteenth century, hospitals became specialized for certain diseases and patient groups, with many catering to particular religious and ethnic populations. They could also be differentiated based on structure, financing, and care objectives. For instance, municipal and county hospitals, which relied on government assistance, offered a full range of acute and chronic care management to the poor. However, market considerations were increasingly shaping hospitals, as they began to rely more heavily on patients' payments. By the early twentieth century, profit-generating hospitals had appeared, operated by physicians and corporations. They were in most cases small surgery centers that treated the wealthy.[6]

Medical education and training became integrated into hospitals during the late nineteenth and early twentieth centuries, as medical practice actively embraced science and research. Elite voluntary hospitals offering acute care management were the first to have direct ties to medical schools; many were the precursors to teaching hospitals. During this period of transformation and growth, one of the first academic medical centers, Johns Hopkins Hospital, opened on May 7, 1889, uniting education, research, and patient care. Johns Hopkins, a wealthy Quaker businessman, had endowed the hospital and required that it "provide for the indigent sick of this city and its environs, without regard to sex, age, or color, who may require surgical or medical treatment."[7] This guiding principle represented a pivotal shift in medicine and hospitals: all patients were welcome to receive care in the same institution, not just either the impoverished or the wealthy. Medical schools and hospitals, which were largely dedicated to training nurses and surgeons,[8] exponentially increased from just a few in the late nineteenth century to over one thousand by 1910. Surgical care emerged as particularly prestigious and lucrative. A greater number of patients were seeking care in hospitals, creating another significant shift in care delivery: hospitals began to limit patient stays for acute periods of illness rather than provide the long-term care that had been the original care model, which was largely derived from the almshouse. During this time, along with development of a training logic, the market logic continued to grow more prominent as hospitals capitalized on financial opportunities borne out of training hospitals.

With transformations in care delivery, hospital budgets rose considerably and charitable donations quickly became insufficient to sustain operations. This required not only a financial restructuring but a general reorganization of care delivery. Administrative needs grew more complex, and authority and power became divided, with physicians now just one group dictating the structuring of care. Proper institutional and financial management was increasingly vital to the hospital's well-being, resulting in a system that was never fully integrated under a single governing or administrative body but rather representative of the multiple critical institutional logics it comprised. This complex organizational structuring has remained a central feature of hospitals in the US, perhaps nowhere more so than in academic medical centers.

Academic medical centers stand out in the current health care landscape for several reasons. First, they tend to see highly complex patients as well as patients with varied financial resources. This diverse patient population affects the clinical environment, giving rise to complicated dilemmas that trainees must learn to address. Second, the responsibility of training future physicians structures care delivery in a specific way, unlike non-teaching hospitals, which offer a much more straightforward delivery model: care tends to be expedited because patients only see attending physicians; important elements of training, such as morning rounds, are absent. In contrast, in academic medical centers patients are frequently seen by a medical team made up of trainees (medical students, interns, and residents) and a supervisor (the attending physician). The structuring of care is inherently different because institutions like PMC must adhere to accreditation requirements that involve medical education, clinical treatment, and research expectations and guidelines. Patients are seen by medical teams through organized morning rounds, which are essential to both care and education:

> The team walks the floor of the medical unit . . . where each patient represents a "classroom episode" of teaching and learning. One of the physicians-in-training . . . presents to the team that patient's history,

laboratory testing, and diagnostic imaging results, as well as a differential diagnosis of possible disease entities that could explain the patient's illness and reason for admission. . . . A discussion then ensues . . . of the most likely diagnoses and best treatment options.[9]

It is not surprising that, because of their pedagogical value, morning rounds can take quite a bit of time (sometimes lasting the entire morning at PMC). While an essential dimension of care delivery, prolonged rounds can also lead to financial consequences for the hospital, such as delays of care, which may not manifest as acutely in non-teaching settings.

From their historical beginnings to their contemporary forms, academic medical centers are a prime example of institutional environments altered by countervailing institutional logics. As physicians encounter conflicts and dilemmas on the clinical wards, they realize that what is considered the best course of action for one institutional logic is frequently not the best for another. This prompts the question: How do physicians juggle the different institutional logics and how do they make care decisions when faced with conflicting pressures and goals? Chapters 3 through 5 will explore these issues empirically, illustrating the conflicts at play and the unintended consequences that stem from physicians' ultimate decisions. In the following sections of this chapter, I lay out the distinct dimensions and dilemmas of the multiple institutional logics found at Pacific Medical Center.

ADHERING TO THE HEALTH LOGIC: THE PROFESSION'S OVERARCHING MORAL IMPERATIVE

Generally, all hospitals and health care practitioners operate under the health logic, striving to "do no harm." Historically, however, this has not always been the case. The latter half of the twentieth century saw unfortunate incidents at US hospitals that revealed an institutional failure to fulfill the responsibility of caring for the acutely ill, mainly in the form of transferring indigent patients to other institutions to avoid financial responsibility for them. In response, the 1986 Emergency Medical Treatment and Labor Act was passed to prohibit hospitals from "dumping" patients. It mandated that all hospital emergency departments examine any patient coming through their doors and stabilize and treat all acutely ill patients regardless of financial status (once stabilized, they could be transferred). Accordingly, all patients who enter the Emergency Department at Pacific Medical Center must be evaluated before any care decisions can be made. While intended to preserve the health logic, this critical legislation is far less straightforward than simply ensuring that all individuals, regardless of ability to pay, are given the acute care they need. Thus, although "do no harm" remains the overarching logic of clinical decisions at PMC, actual decisions rarely fall into a single category or represent just one institutional logic.

What does adhering to the health logic and providing quality care actually entail? Numerous health metrics are frequently calculated to determine care quality. Two of the most common are morbidity and mortality. Others are safety (e.g., patient falls) and hospital-acquired infection. Pacific Medical Center successfully meets, at minimum, the national average (though often performing better than the average) for a variety of hospital performance metrics, including hospital-acquired infection, surgery problems, error prevention protocols, and best safety practices.

In recent years, hospitals have moved beyond what are deemed to be objective or standardized metrics of health and safety, and now focus on patients: specifically, how well hospitals and health care professionals provide patient-centered care, which is often measured by patient satisfaction. Patient-centered care "fosters interactions in which clinicians and patients engage in two-way sharing of information; explore patients' values and preferences; help patients and their families make clinical decisions; facilitate access to appropriate care; and enable patients to follow through with often difficult behavioral changes needed to maintain or improve health."[10] Often used to assess physician and care quality, patient satisfaction determines whether the "physician has provided comfort, emotional support, education, and considered the patient's perspective in the synthesis of the clinical decision making process."[11] The inclusion of patients and families in medical decision-making has become synonymous with patient-centered care and is a strong predictor of satisfied patients. Studies have found that shared decision-making results in patients' increased knowledge, more accurate risk perceptions, reduced internal conflict about decisions, and greater likelihood of receiving care aligned with their values.[12]

Financial incentives reflect the emphasis on patient satisfaction. In 2011 the Centers for Medicare and Medicaid Services finalized a new reimbursement method that adjusts payments based on patient satisfaction scores.[13] Pacific Medical Center regularly administers patient satisfaction surveys and offers various amenities on the inpatient wards (e.g., private rooms, made-to-order meals). The Internal Medicine Service is committed to patient-centered care, with attending physicians in particular spending time with patients and families, making sure that they feel heard and included in decisions, particularly about discharge.

To this point, I have focused on the contradictory aspects of the institutional logics and the arduous task of reconciling them when making care determinations. However, these logics also align with one another when the practices and objectives of one meet the demands of another. For instance, patient-centered indicators of care quality (and the health logic) are undeniably linked to the health care legal logic. It is hardly coincidental that the emphasis on patient-centered care and patient satisfaction emerged shortly after the rise in health care litigation and malpractice lawsuits in the US. Medical malpractice was first seen in the 1840s and became increasingly visible during the twentieth and the early twenty-first centuries. The United States stands out as a nation where lawsuits against health care professionals are incredibly common, contributing to its high health care spending.[14] The American Medical Association reports that two-thirds of US states are experiencing a "malpractice crisis."[15]

"Defensive medicine" is commonly used to characterize the tendency of providers to overtreat patients, bending to their preferences and requests even when the care is unnecessary or excessive.[16] This relatively recent phenomenon stems from major transformations in the experiences of physicians over the course of the twentieth century. The first half of the century found physicians experiencing professional dominance[17] during what is often characterized as the "golden age of medicine."[18] In contrast, in the second half of the century they were increasingly embroiled in legal battles as reports of medical negligence and physicians placing financial gain above patient welfare were highly publicized. This period ushered in an era of patient-centered care accelerated by this growing distrust of physicians and medicine.[19] Gone was the era of paternalism[20] and in its place were much more informed patient-consumers unafraid to make demands regarding their care and take legal action if not satisfied.[21] With legal concerns featuring prominently in the minds of health care providers, the United States saw the rise of defensive medicine.[22] Now physicians increasingly make decisions based on litigation risk and patients are routinely subjected to unnecessary interventions, which can have physical, emotional, and financial repercussions.

Consequently, publicized malpractice lawsuits and shifts in patient identities have made the legal logic fundamental in health care settings. Health care professionals say that litigation is glaringly featured in their daily work. The highly litigious nature of the US patient population has had a direct impact on physician autonomy, impinged on the patient-physician relationship, and resulted in greater professional dissatisfaction, collectively shaping how health care professionals approach care delivery.[23] IM physicians at Pacific Medical Center are cognizant of their vulnerable legal status—particularly attending physicians, who are legally responsible for the patients on the IM wards.

Another important feature of an institution's health logic is interspecialty care, which is increasingly equated with improvements in health outcomes and patient satisfaction. Academic medical centers like PMC are touted for the highly specialized care they offer: interspecialty care is routine and expected. For instance, Michael, a 22-year-old man living with Crohn's disease and opiate dependency, came to the Emergency Department at Pacific Medical Center with osteomyelitis,[24] malnourishment, and an ulcer. He was quickly admitted to the Internal Medicine Service and within the first twenty-four hours of his stay, his medical team had consulted with Surgery, Interventional Radiology, Infectious Disease, Gastroenterology, and Psychiatry. Before Michael left the hospital, Nutrition and Rheumatology were also brought onboard, resulting in eight different teams coordinating his care. While the heavy reliance on interspecialty care is a universal phenomenon, the fact that Internal Medicine is a generalist service further contributes to specialist use: because internists have broad knowledge of various adult diseases and conditions rather than expertise in specific illnesses, organ systems, or procedures, they are expected to call on specialists to treat their patients.

Interspecialty care is a direct consequence of the increased specialization of medicine and the financial profits associated with it. Specialists are expensive—they generate high costs. Merely calling a consultant triggers a fee. Furthermore, by bringing additional physicians onboard, there is greater likelihood of patients undergoing increased testing, procedures, and scans, accelerating inpatient spending. Specialists are also increasingly necessary from a legal perspective, contributing to the practice of defensive medicine. Each consultant called on to coordinate patient care is perceived as bringing in more expertise and in turn, offering better care to patients. It is important to note that interspecialty care is driven not solely by the nature of the medical profession or the profit motive but also by patient demands for better care, which often means more experts and more care.

Because practitioners strive for the health logic by ensuring patient satisfaction and routinely engaging specialists at Pacific Medical Center, inpatient dilemmas arise. As quality care has become synonymous with both health outcome measures and patient-centered metrics, physicians must not only address patients' physical needs but also ensure that their experiences in the hospital are satisfying. As discussed earlier, at PMC the commitment to patient satisfaction and its inevitable relationship with defensive medicine are evident in numerous ways: from physicians' deference to patients' care and discharge requests to the private rooms and amenities made available. The unintended consequence is that sometimes patients prefer not to leave the comfort and safety of the hospital and physicians go along.[25] Patients who remain in the hospital without an acute medical need are especially problematic for several of the hospital's institutional logics. From a market standpoint, it is expensive to house patients unnecessarily. From a health standpoint, patients can become sick or injured during their hospital stay or they occupy beds that others in need of inpatient care should occupy. And from a training standpoint, these patients offer little new. Thus, in an effort to meet the expectations of good care, there are inevitable trade-offs that compromise the institutional logics, because what is ultimately best for one patient is not necessarily what is best for other patients, trainees, or the hospital itself.

Interspecialty care can also compromise the hospital's market logic. Medical workups by consultants normally take time to complete and interpret, resulting in costly delays of care and extended hospital stays. The more individuals involved in patient care, the higher the obstacles to consensus on a treatment plan. Ineffective communication and ensuing disagreements lead to further expensive delays of care (and discharge). To combat delays, and their financial penalties, IM physicians learn to preemptively run tests such as blood work or begin paperwork for scans and procedures that they expect the consultant will request. This strategy is contingent on the IM team's ability to anticipate the specialists' demands.

For example, a 45-year-old lung transplant patient had been admitted to the hospital with a persistent cough and shortness of breath. During morning rounds, the IM team decided it would be best to call for an Infectious Disease (ID) consult because the patient was immunosuppressed. The attending told the team, "We should start the full ID workup. They always request [it] so we can just start it now." The interns and the resident agreed. The attending continued: "It isn't because *we* think it's necessary but we have seen enough times that this is what ID wants." Preemptive workups are valuable because, instead of waiting for the ID consultant to make an official request for lab work, the IM team expedited delivery of the information to the specialist. Such strategies are in response to the unintended consequences of clinical decisions made on the wards and reveal the complexities of medical decision-making amid conflicting institutional pressures and goals. IM physicians quickly learn that the health logic looks different from what they may have believed it to be in medical school, and the ability to best meet its demands require trainees to learn how to successfully navigate the institution's market, legal, and training logics as well.

––––––––––––

THE INEVITABLE NEED FOR THE MARKET LOGIC IN HEALTH CARE

The market logic is arguably the most controversial of the institutional logics in the US health care system. The sociocultural image of practitioners striving to do no harm precisely requires that they ignore the financial implications of the care they provide. However, this is no longer possible and in many ways it is unadvisable for financial considerations to be wholly ignored, as revealed by the tale of the Allegheny Health, Education, and Research Foundation (AHERF). On July 21, 1998, AHERF, one of the largest health care providers in Pennsylvania, filed for bankruptcy, reporting a debt of $1.3 billion and losses of $1 million on a daily basis.[26] Making national headlines, the collapse of AHERF was the "nation's largest nonprofit health care bankruptcy and second-largest overall . . . [signaling] the end of the largest statewide integrated delivery system in Pennsylvania [and] the largest medical school in the country."[27] The Allegheny bankruptcy has become a cautionary tale of medical mismanagement and poor financial decision-making. Often the tendency is to focus on patients' experiences with bankruptcy due to the high costs of care.[28] However, AHERF is just one example of the importance of proper financial management in hospitals themselves. While not on as large a scale as the AHERF collapse, hospital closures are common across the country and are particularly concerning in rural regions. Five percent of the nation's rural hospitals have closed since 2010.[29] Obstetric care has "faced even starker cutbacks as rural hospitals calculate the hard math of survival, weighing the cost of providing 24/7 delivery services against dwindling birthrates, doctor and nursing shortages and falling revenues."[30] As hospitals close their doors or merge[31] to remain viable, patients suffer—some must travel a hundred miles for necessary care[32] and everyone faces higher prices because hospital mergers decrease competition.[33]

Hospitals require proper financial management to keep their doors open: they must run as a business with profit a critical component in their sustainability, and the sustainability of the broader US health care system. Financial considerations and the market logic became especially prominent with the introduction of managed care in the 1970s and health care managerialism in the 1980s,[34] which promoted efficiency and cost containment in the clinical setting to combat excessive, wasteful spending.[35] This entrepreneurial ethos[36] became further evident as profit maximization became embedded in medical decision-making[37] and health care became increasingly rationed; physicians were expected to regularly calculate costs when administering care (e.g., time spent with patients, costs of medical interventions).[38] Health care organizations and professionals in turn became progressively more accountable[39] to the singular goal of constraining costs without compromising care.[40]

Since the late twentieth century, hospitals have been under pressure to reduce costs—specifically unnecessary spending, frequently referred to as medical waste.[41] In 2011 failures of care delivery (such as poor execution) cost $102–$154 billion, failures in care coordination (e.g., unnecessary hospital readmissions) cost $25–$45 billion, overtreatment cost $158–$226 billion, and administrative complexity cost $107–$389 billion.[42] A 2019 *JAMA* article reviewing literature published from January 2012 to May 2019 presents similar, if not greater, ranges, with medical waste estimated to cost $760–$935 billion annually.[43] This preventable expenditure is not a new issue but one that has plagued the health care system for many decades and one that has been met with various professional and organizational solutions.

In the late twentieth century, two new employment opportunities developed in the health care setting. One was the job of hospitalist introduced in 1996 by Dr. Robert Wachter and Dr. Lee Goldman. The other was the job of care coordination, primarily conducted by nurse discharge planners. The Society of Hospital Medicine (SHM)[44] defines a hospitalist as "dedicated to the delivery of comprehensive medical care to hospitalized patients."[45] Previously, most general internists split their time between office and hospital visits. However, reimbursement policies established in the 1970s discouraged inpatient work with minimal payback; work that could be performed as outpatient care was preferred.[46] As primary care physicians dedicated more time to office work, they were less available for inpatient care. The result was extended hospital stays and rising inpatient costs. The proposed solution was generalist physicians dedicating their time to inpatient care. By working in a single setting, hospitalists are more accustomed to the conditions of hospitalized patients—improving quality of care while also being more attuned to the complexities of hospital care delivery and thus expediting care and decreasing health care spending.[47] Indeed, studies have confirmed that the adoption of hospitalists has led to reductions in costs, decreased lengths of stay, and increased efficiency—all without a drop in quality.[48]

Care coordination teams are dedicated to discharge planning. Since the 1970s, there had been an emphasis across US hospitals to shorten hospital stays to reduce costs. Decreasing lengths of stay were further motivated by the introduction of diagnosis-related groups (DRGs) in 1983.[49] DRGs changed the reimbursement system, with hospitals now paid per diagnosis rather than for all services performed. As a result, there was a greater push to shorten stays to minimize financial losses for the hospital. One solution was the discharge planner. The goals of discharge planning are not only to decrease delays but also to ensure that rehabilitation and outpatient care are well established to prevent readmission.[50]

Although some studies have indicated a reduction in health care costs,[51] the hospitalist and the discharge planner have been largely insufficient as health care costs have ballooned from approximately $247 billion in 1980[52] to $3.5 trillion in 2017.[53] Nonetheless, like hospitals across the United States, Pacific Medical Center has embraced hospitalists and care coordination teams in efforts to reduce inpatient spending. Hospitalists predominantly run the IM wards. Furthermore, in the early part of my research, case managers were assigned to each IM team and actively participated in morning rounds by overseeing patient discharge and other financial and social issues. Recognizing the complexities of the discharge process, the Internal Medicine Service conducts multidisciplinary rounds in the afternoon with the attending, resident, case manager, social worker, physical therapy specialists, and other practitioners who have had (or may have) an impact on a patient's discharge date. These rounds are in place specifically to discuss current and potential discharge problems.

In the pursuit of health logic goals, hospitals and practitioners inevitably face unintended financial consequences. Academic medical centers incur greater financial losses because they tend to provide more safety-net or unreimbursed care, emergency and intensive care, and mental health care compared with other institutions.[54] While policies and legislation like the Emergency Medical Treatment and Labor Act are essential in protecting patients' rights, hospitals face the financial burden of caring for those who cannot pay. Pacific Medical Center provides a great deal of care to homeless patients, who have extended hospital stays because, even if they have been stabilized, they have nowhere to go.[55] Furthermore, even nonhomeless patients, because many of them have complex needs, often cannot be discharged to their homes but must be transferred to skilled nursing facilities and other centers that offer higher levels of care. Lack of available beds in these settings leads to costly extended hospital stays as well.

Financial losses generate much of the unnecessary spending that has been extensively discussed when evaluating the US health care system. To offset some of them, IM physicians quickly learn the importance of the social dimensions of patient care and to be prepared to navigate the unexpected nonmedical dilemmas they give rise to. Successful navigation typically goes hand in hand with early preparation, especially when dealing with hospital discharge management. The motto at PMC is that discharge planning should begin on day one. Trainees are regularly reminded of this when the attending asks them at patient admission, "Does the patient have any potential dispo issues?" This simple question forces them to articulate all of the medical and social issues that may impede getting the patient out the door. Trainees appreciate these reminders to plan ahead because as one second-year resident frankly stated, "The approach to discharge is *day one*. If you wait on it, you get *screwed*."

Ironically, market-driven decisions inevitably lead to greater financial conse-quences for the hospital as well. As noted earlier, case managers equip physi-cians with financial information on their patients; they know the restrictions of particular health insurance plans and the affordable options available based on insurance status. However, over the course of my research I saw budgetary constraints and lack of personnel result in inconsistent use of case managers. The consequence of limited resources and turnover of personnel was that multiple teams shared a single case manager, who was juggling forty or more patients and was physically unable to participate in morning rounds. Case managers made every effort to communicate regularly with physicians, but their inconsistent attendance at rounds inevitably affected care delivery. Without them, there were issues of outpatient care coordination, insurance coverage, and hospital discharge that attendings were unsure of how to han-dle. Thus they would need to contact case managers after rounds, before proceeding with a care plan, causing costly delays of care and discharge.

Nights and weekends are another instance of financially driven decisions having consequences: there are fewer people staffing the hospital during these times (including providers and case managers), leading to delays in care. While weekend closures and fewer staff on hand are common in most business settings, they can be problematic in the hospital because no one can predict or control when someone will become acutely ill or injured and need medical attention. There are individuals and protocols in place for emergent situations, however in most other cases, services and providers are lacking, meaning once again delays of care. A second-year Emergency Medicine resident explained the dilemma that arises: "On the wards, when we have patients [with] gastrointestinal issues, it's common knowledge that it's very hard to get a gastrointestinal consultant in the middle of the night unless the patient truly is hemodynamically unstable," so the patient must wait until the next day to receive specialized care. An attending also pointed to the ramifications of weekend closures for the hospital:

> I would say the big issues have more to do with the fact that the hospital doesn't operate on the weekend . . . so we can't get diagnostic tests on the weekends that we might want, or procedures on the weekends that we might want, or discharge people on the weekends. If we could operate on the weekends the way we do during the week, we could really shorten people's length of stay.

From an administration standpoint, the costs of operating with full services presumably outweigh the costs associated with delays of care and discharge from the hospital due to lack of staffing during nonbusiness hours. Nevertheless, the hospital still incurs costs that could be avoided. As might be expected, financial dilemmas arise constantly on the clinical wards at Pacific Medical Center. Physicians learn as they garner more experience in the inpatient setting to recognize when financial considerations should drive care decisions and when financial losses are simply a necessary by-product of the care decisions they must make.

THE DILEMMAS OF TRAINING

The commitment and practices adopted to train physicians often run counter to the objectives and goals of hospitals. For instance, in order to effectively educate them, novice physicians typically provide the bulk of care, which may occasionally undermine the health logic. Inevitably mistakes are made by interns and residents[56] that are simply a result of the learning process. Furthermore, patients may find themselves in prolonged limbo, as attendings give trainees the time and space to work out diagnoses and treatment plans primarily on their own. Such uncertainty can have ill effects on a patient's emotional state and lead to greater dissatisfaction with care. Indeed, some studies have indicated concerns about compromised care at the hands of physicians-in-training, yet others have shown that teaching institutions typically have low morbidity and mortality rates compared with non-teaching institutions.[57] These improved outcomes have largely been attributed to high-quality practitioners, cutting-edge research, and access to new technologies.

Along with its impact on the health logic, teaching is frequently at odds with the institution's financial goals. The Association of American Medical Colleges reports that teaching hospitals incur more than $17 billion in direct training costs each year. Studies have reported that they use more resources and have higher expenditures due to educational needs than non-teaching institutions.[58] Some of the conversations I had with IM physicians at Pacific Medical Center resonated with these findings. During morning rounds one day, the attending and resident discussed the costs of tests and workups for a patient with pancreatic cancer. The attending said, "These tests and workups are great for academic interest. Especially for someone under one year in the program," but he said that they translated into astronomical patient expenditure. The resident agreed: "For instance, the whole anemia workup. It costs so much more when completed on inpatient rather than on an outpatient, and it doesn't change our management here . . . we just automatically do the workup, which is good from an academic perspective." This exchange revealed the persistent tension between effective teaching and cost-conscious care delivery at PMC.

Dr. Brandon, Director of Residency Training at PMC, reflected on this tension:

> We . . . train our residents and housestaff . . . to be very, very thorough. So when you're rounding . . . on the wards with the teams, they come up with hypotheses about what's going on with the patient. And the attending says, "Okay, that's fine." So you've got two or three things, but what about this and what about that, and what about x, y, and z. You know, by the end of rounds you have a longer list of potential problems that have to be excluded. And what we always encourage is that . . . the housestaff use the history and the physical exam as the strongest and the most cost-effective tools for ruling things out. But very often, if you bring up an

issue that . . . involves checking some tests, that will drive up the costs further because the housestaff will order a liver panel or . . . a viral serology panel to rule out something that you brought up in rounds.

Given Internal Medicine's global perspective, interns and residents must consider all possible causes of a particular set of symptoms and conditions, which can require extensive resource use for teaching purposes.

Dr. Brandon discussed the conflicting financial pressures and the impact they have on medical training:

Academic medical centers are under pressure to save money and to rein in costs. So . . . you have the situation . . . where you're teaching trainees and you want to be thorough and you want to encourage them to . . . in essence, rule in and rule out their hypotheses. . . . At the same time, you have this pressure to get the patients in and out as quickly as possible . . . so you know somebody can continue their workup as an outpatient [and] you know you want to discharge them as soon as possible and not only discharge them but discharge them before noon . . . so that you can turn the room around and bring in the next patient. And there's no question this has impacted the housestaff. The residents see this and . . . begin to wonder[if this is]priority learning and education or is it generating income. . . . It's a huge conflict because at the same time, if you're not a cost-effective and efficiently run medical center, you're not going to be in business for very long and you're not going to have residents to teach. So we find as attendings that probably our single biggest dilemma is striking a balance between those two things—where you want to be able to . . . [say to] residents and housestaff . . . "Look, this is the time when you are learning to be a doctor: we want you to be cost-effective but we also want you to be thorough and humanistic and use physical diagnostic skills that you have learned appropriately, and not overorder tests. And you have to do that all within two and a half days because . . . we know from research that patients with this particular diagnosis—usually the national mean—spend two and a half days in the hospital. If you keep them here longer, you're in essence failing as a practitioner."

Mixed messages create dilemmas for attendings, who must successfully train young physicians but prevent financially irresponsible care. Unfortunately, this can lead to disenchanted trainees who question whether their current role is to advance their skills and continue their education or to simply learn to make care decisions that meet the hospital's bottom line.

The claim that teaching hospitals incur greater health care costs are not uniformly supported.[59] Furthermore, hospitalists have been found to lower costs in teaching hospitals while improving the trainee experience.[60] As discussed previously, PMC has embraced hospitalists, giving them primary control over the Internal Medicine Service. Furthermore, through regular communication during the day with case management and discharge planners, care is expedited and physicians learn about the various financial and bureaucratic dimensions to care delivery.

Notably, it is not simply learning itself that results in expensive care; the structuring of care in teaching hospitals exacerbates health care spending as well. For instance, the scheduling of morning rounds at PMC is directly influenced by the ACGME (Accreditation Council for Graduate Medical Education) requirement to have trainees first meet for Morning Report, when housestaff gather together to discuss interesting patient cases. The timing of morning rounds has spillover effects: they frequently start at nine-thirty and last until noon or even one, so orders for tests, procedures, and consultants may not be placed until the afternoon. This dramatically decreases the chance that particular tests or consults will be carried out on the same day. Fortunately, as trainees progress through their residency they develop strategies to offset the consequences of lengthy rounds. They learn to momentarily step away from the team to initiate a consult or schedule a procedure. It is especially vital to call consultants as soon as possible because the point of contact is usually consulting fellows, who must *also* confer with *their* supervising attending before any official medical orders or treatment plans can be carried out.

Preemptive paperwork for procedures is another strategy trainees learn in order to advance care delivery. There are times when the consulting fellow verbally indicates that a procedure may be necessary pending test results or discussion with the specialist attending. If the procedure is indicated, the paperwork will already have been started, expediting the process.

The costs of medical training remain controversial, with some calling for a change in the medical training model[61] and others arguing that the benefits of the current model far outweigh its drawbacks. Opponents believe that failure to control spending will leave academic medical centers with a precarious future: they simply will not be viable in the long term. Proponents, like Dr. David Silbersweig, chairman of the Department of Psychiatry and codirector of the Institute for the Neurosciences at Brigham and Women's Hospital in Boston, have argued that what is gained from teaching hospitals is well worth their costs:

> But how does one measure the incidence of getting the diagnosis right (let alone the costs, not just in unnecessary tests, of not getting it right)? How does one quantify the expertise that enables academic medical doctors and teams to treat the most complex, acute, or refractory cases in a manner beyond the case mix index? How does one capture the reason why physicians in other settings routinely refer patients to teaching hospitals when they can't figure out what is going on, when there are complications, or when they have run out of treatment options?[62]

Dr. Silbersweig echoes the common belief that training hospitals preserve the best of medicine: top-notch care that has a profound impact on health outcomes and lives. High resource utilization and other costs of training are necessary to ensure that quality care is available to anyone who needs it.

Market, legal, and training concerns deeply influence how IM physicians at Pacific Medical Center make clinical decisions. However, these decisions are frequently rationalized as a result of the hospital's health logic, with little mention of the market, legal, and training logics. For example, I observed IM physicians frequently telling their team that a consultant would be unnecessary and would not improve a patient's health outcomes or dramatically alter patient care, yet they still called in a specialist, emphasizing the value of specialty expertise. Sometimes physicians would knowingly discharge a severely ill yet underresourced patient to a lower-quality facility, citing the financial impact of keeping them in the hospital on their overall health and well-being. Yet the same physicians also invoked the health logic and the importance of patient welfare to justify keeping many stable patients despite insurance companies urging discharge, choosing to risk incurring a financial penalty for the hospital. Collectively, such examples show flexibility in the health logic and "doing no harm," revealing how IM physicians capitalize on the moral polysemy of the health logic in negotiating conflicting institutional logics and pressures. This results in moral evaluations and clinical decisions made on a case-by-case basis and divergent patient outcomes as well as distinct consequences for both health care practitioners and the hospital.

CONCLUSION

Since their inception in the late eighteenth and early nineteenth centuries and their transformation during the nineteenth and twentieth centuries, all hospitals have had to contend with the challenges and dilemmas of multiple, conflicting institutional logics that are essential to the sustainability of the hospital. At Pacific Medical Center, the health, market, legal, and training logics deeply affect the experiences of physicians on the IM wards. They create a working environment that is a microcosm of the broader health care system. One particularly important transformation in health care has been commodification and bureaucratization requiring third-party involvement, which serves some institutional logics better than others.

Physicians-in-training experience the interference of third parties primarily through the medical record, which has become a site of contradictory institutional logics that must be carefully negotiated. The following chapter explores how trainees learn to use the medical record on the wards and avoid the high stakes of improper use, which can threaten health outcomes and lead to expensive consequences for the patient and the hospital.

3 | NOTATION

Jessica, a white woman, was diagnosed with Crohn's disease at 23 years of age. A year later, she arrived at the Emergency Department (ED) at Pacific Medical Center with worsening abdominal pain and decreased appetite. In the ED, she underwent a CT scan of her abdomen and pelvis and was admitted to the Internal Medicine Service. Upon assessment of the scan, the primary care team was uncertain as to whether Jessica was experiencing a Crohn's flare, a mild obstruction, a fistula, or a polyp. Within the first twenty-four hours of her hospital stay, Gastroenterology had been consulted and was following the patient. The morning after she had been admitted, the intern assigned to Jessica's case informed the team during morning rounds that he had contacted the colorectal consultant, who was now also caring for the patient. As the team contemplated the patient's treatment plan, Dr. Lee, the attending, suggested one option: "Hit the patient with a higher dose of steroids and if she worsens, take her to surgery." He asked the team, "Are we doing a step-up—start with steroids and then go up in treatment—or a top-down—hit hard first with TNF inhibitors and then taper down?" The resident responded that patients like Jessica tend to be hit hard when hospitalized but usually are "already on PO medications at home, and this patient isn't on medications so that makes her potentially a bit different in terms of treatment plan." Dr. Lee nodded and told the team to wait and ask Gastroenterology (GI) before proceeding.

Over two days, the team was able to determine that Jessica had a Crohn's flare and a mild obstruction. Unfortunately, she had not had a bowel movement in the last twenty-four hours, had begun experiencing increased eye swelling and eye pain, and had black urine output. The intern had ordered a urinalysis and Ophthalmology had been called in. After an eye exam, the Ophthalmology consultant suggested putting the patient on methylprednisone drops. Because of her distended and painful abdomen, Radiology had also been contacted and had noted "signs of small bowel dilation."

During the following day's morning rounds, one intern reported a conflict between two consultants on Jessica's team. Surgery felt that her primary acute issues had been addressed and she was stabilized so she could be transferred to an outside hospital. GI was not comfortable with the proposed discharge and wanted to hold her. The resident interjected and explained to the team that this discussion of a potential transfer had arisen because of Jessica's insurance coverage: she would not be able to stay long term at Pacific Medical Center. One of the medical students also confirmed that the patient's insurer was on the team's case: he had received a call from them. After a review of her record, they considered Jessica stabilized and wanted her transferred from Pacific Medical Center to another hospital.

"What is GI's concern regarding transfer?" Dr. Lee asked. The resident explained that GI was worried about the quality of care and PMC's distance from Anders, the hospital Jessica would be transferred to. Furthermore, Jessica hated it there. The resident explained that she had spoken with the insurance company and it had offered one more day, but she was not sure how much more "we can push back and whether we will get any additional days." The attending sighed; he had heard concerns about Anders and was "certain that she would receive better care at PMC." The resident nodded in agreement but noted: "We *also* don't want to leave her with a huge bill either." The attending replied: "Yes…well, she is improving and there is no urgent need for a procedure with Surgery," which meant that she would have to be transferred no matter what. As the IM team had expected, Jessica was transferred to Anders because there was no acute medical reason for prolonging her stay at PMC.

The exchange between physicians about Jessica's treatment protocol, and the ultimate decision to transfer her to Anders, reveal how IM physicians engage in moral polysemy to explain clinical decisions that are fundamentally driven by financial constraints at Pacific Medical Center. While cases like Allegheny Health in Pennsylvania reveal the high stakes of mismanaging the market logic (Chapter 2), Jessica's case highlights the inevitable trade-offs in market considerations: Jessica was sent to a health care facility that the PMC physicians readily acknowledged would provide inferior care and one where Jessica did not want to go. This vignette reminds us of the contradictory objectives of the market and health logics in health care and the fact that clinical decisions shaped by financial limitations can appear to be a direct violation of the health logic: the transfer decision was not in the best "health" interest of the patient. However, to make sense of it, the IM team emphasized both the financial liability that would inevitably befall Jessica and her stable condition to justify her transfer from a patient welfare perspective.

This juggling of costs and benefits when making medical decisions resonates with Altomonte's (2020) findings on varied discharge decisions for elderly patients from a postacute care unit, where ethical, legal, and economic pressures result in conflicting organizational objectives. Drawing on different definitions of independent aging, the staff rationalize choices to hold certain patients while quickly discharging others. Altomonte (2020) explains this process as an "exploiting of the moral polysemy of independent aging," which allows multiple meanings of independent aging to make sense of these decisions.[1] Similarly, the care plan for Jessica is a key example of how IM physicians at Pacific Medical Center exploit the moral polysemy of the health logic to make sense of situational clinical decisions they are forced to make.

Such difficult determinations are not a rare occurrence at PMC; countless times I saw underinsured and uninsured patients transferred out of the hospital if they did not have acute medical needs. Even with insured patients, IM physicians encountered challenges to care decisions and denials of coverage by third-party payers via the medical record. The IM team typically catches wind of financial issues when the insurer starts calling the hospital upon review of a patient's medical record. This interference is a reminder of the critical role the medical record plays in care delivery—as sociologists have demonstrated it is not simply a legal document carefully delineating a patient's medical history and current health status but also a social object that shapes interactions (and communication) between providers and other parties.[2] Sociologists call it a formal organizing tool of medical information, favoring particular forms of information and actively shaping how care is provided. For instance, since insurance companies are not at the hospital overseeing care and interacting with patients and providers, the medical record becomes the only way they can make coverage assessments. Proper medical documentation is thus vital to ensure that patients receive the care they need without being held financially responsible.

Either insurers carefully review the patient's medical record and care plan and then call team members, as happened with Jessica, or the hospital's case management teams communicate determinations of coverage for prescribed treatments, procedures, and lengths of stay. In this way, medical documentation becomes a critical dimension of physician training and education, with multifaceted dilemmas and lessons to be learned. As expected in a training hospital, interns bear the brunt of documentation, learning to properly write orders and chronicle care. While seemingly straightforward, it is not always clear what "proper documentation" and "proper use" entail as it can mean different things in different contexts. Because the information provided in the medical record is used by numerous parties with different objectives, IM physicians are careful about what is documented and how. A predicament for interns in their first year of residency is that their inexperience increases the potential for errors in documentation and its use. Such errors have implications for patient care, hospital finances, and IM physicians themselves, especially from a legal standpoint. The remainder of this chapter explores these varied dilemmas and experiences with medical documentation on the IM wards at Pacific Medical Center.

PROPER USE OF THE MEDICAL RECORD: AN INTERPLAY OF LOGICS

The medical record is "essential to evaluating, ensuring and improving the quality of health care. . . . It improves the coordination and continuity of care, reinforces decision-making capacities, augments staff accountability and achieves more accurate vital statistics."[3] It also communicates information about patients to the "individual practitioner, consultants, third-party payers, lawyers and clinical investigators."[4] At Pacific Medical Center, the medical record structures interactions across physicians, nurses, case managers, insurers, and other health care actors. Its proper documentation and use facilitate efficient care coordination and minimal interactions across these actors via notes, pages, and occasional phone calls. With interactions streamlined, primary care physicians rarely meet with others involved in patient care in real time. According to one resident, "[there are] consultants that I'm meeting face to face for the first time six months in."

In its optimal form, the medical record supports the institution's health, market, and legal logics. Many scholars have championed the role it plays in increasing efficiency, reducing costs, and improving overall care.[5] Embraced by hospitals across the country since the early 2000s, the electronic medical record has been found especially to improve health outcomes and quality of care.[6]

The medical record protects the institution's market logic because insurers make financial assessments that further the goals of managed care: cost containment and efficiency. While these factors inevitably constrain the care decisions physicians make, they also serve as a valuable reminder for them to consider the financial implications of care delivery for both the patient and the hospital. Lastly, the medical record upholds the hospital's legal logic: clear and detailed documentation of each clinical decision and treatment plan protects physicians and the hospital from accusations of medical negligence. Because it is a legal document itself, the medical record leaves physicians vulnerable to litigation, so they learn the importance of careful documentation.

The training logic at PMC complicates experiences with medical documentation. In a teaching hospital, interns, overseen by residents, complete much of the day-to-day documentation, so it is crucial that they learn to do it correctly. Inexperience predictably leads to errors, however, disrupting patient care and leaving patients without necessary treatments. In addition, incorrect documentation can lead to misinformed insurers, whose subsequent financial decision-making may delay care and cause financial losses for the patient and the hospital. Such errors and improper use of the medical record create inefficiencies in care delivery.

"Inefficient care" is a phrase frequently used when discussing the pitfalls of the US health care system, in tandem with "medical waste." Inefficiencies are a major concern for health care professionals, administrators, and policymakers because the system loses billions of dollars annually to avoidable and unnecessary medical waste.[7] A 2013 Institute of Medicine report found that approximately 30 percent of health care spending was due to unnecessary or poorly delivered services that cost nearly $750 billion.[8] At the institutional level, medical waste can take many forms; one in particular is overtreatment, such as repeated tests, and delays, which have been targeted as remarkably expensive dimensions of care delivery. At Pacific Medical Center, IM physicians are attuned to these concerns and strive to avoid care delays and unnecessary procedures that stem from improper medical documentation.

One of the first lessons trainees must learn is *what* to write in the medical record: what information must be included regarding patient care. In instances of denials of coverage, insurance companies typically contact the attending physician or the case manager assigned to the primary care team. Denials halt care, so physicians must then complete additional work (phone calls with insurers, revised notation, and so forth) before care can proceed, leaving patients waiting for needed treatment.

The clinical inexperience of interns juxtaposed with their responsibility for most medical documentation often results in disputes. A case manager explained to me that a key problem is that trainees are often too vague and fail to provide enough detail to prove why the patient should be in the hospital. The attending agreed that trainees' lack of clinical experience results in many disagreements that could have been easily averted or promptly resolved:

> [Financial issues are] very salient at all times, especially since the case manager is telling us about the patient's insurance status—that they are out of network or that the health insurance company has rejected the patient's stay. In these cases, usually all you have to do is change the wording on the hospital notes. Early on in my training, it was unclear what a "justifiable hospital stay"[9] was, but now I know better.

Accordingly, the case manager and the attending physician guide trainees in medical documentation.

Considering the implications of improper medical documentation, attending physicians invest much time teaching trainees what to write. They frequently offer a verbal outline of exactly *how* a condition should be

documented, exposing trainees to the "language" of insurance companies—
the specific terms that health insurance companies read as billable conditions
and therapies. There is often a disconnect, however, between insurers' billable
language and the biomedical terms physicians use in everyday practice. Effective communication between physicians and insurers is therefore contingent
on trainees learning the language. For example, once during morning rounds,
the attending physician explained to the team the right and wrong way to
document their 63-year-old patient's urosepsis, an infection of the blood
caused by a urinary tract infection. Upon examining the woman, the attending found that she was experiencing worsening right flank pain, a cough,
and little urine output that was cloudy. After leaving the patient's room,
the attending discussed with the resident and interns how to document her
condition. He told the interns not to notate the condition as "urosepsis [but
as] sepsis from a urinary source" to ensure that the insurer would not dispute
the medical assessment. He explained that the condition is often incorrectly
written as urosepsis, which the insurer does not recognize as billable. To
the frustration of trainees, while they may have correctly documented the
condition from a medical standpoint, their notation would not meet the
insurer's criteria and so coverage would be denied.

Along with what to write, trainees must also learn *where* to write particular pieces of information, usually orders, in the record. Case management
is especially helpful for how to do this. For instance, an 81-year-old woman
living with advanced Alzheimer's needed a walker in order to be discharged.
After evaluating the patient during morning rounds, the case manager presented the resident with an order for the walker, which would be included
in the patient's record. As the resident scanned the order, she glanced at the
case manager confused and asked, "Do I write [the order] here?" pointing to
a section of the record. The case manager responded, "Yes. . . . I can handle
the rest." She said she would have the walker brought to the patient prior to
her discharge.

In addition to what to write and where, the logistics of medical documentation—specifically *when* to write—is a critical lesson for trainees. It
is particularly important at Pacific Medical Center, which runs at overca-
pacity and whose patient population is highly complex, needing numerous
procedures, tests, and specialists—all requiring timely documentation and

placement of orders for care to move forward. The ability to expedite this process is directly impacted by the structuring of care delivery at teaching hospitals. During morning rounds, the IM team typically decides whether additional tests, procedures, or consultations are needed or the patient is stable enough to be discharged.

Early in my research, when case managers rounded with the medical team and the team primarily used paper, the case manager would compile all of the records in large binders and bring them along during rounds so that trainees could complete time-sensitive notation, such as placing an order for a specific procedure or a consultant, immediately rather than wait until rounds concluded. The earlier that order was placed, the greater the likelihood that the patient would receive the test or be seen by a consultant that day. In turn, trainees quickly learned which information was time-sensitive and must be written in the record without delay, and which could be input later. For instance, one patient was ready to be discharged and merely needed transportation. The case manager told an intern that an ambulance needed to be scheduled for midafternoon that day in order for the patient to be discharged. She instructed the intern to write *"right now,"* meaning ten o'clock, to ensure that the ambulance would be secured.

Through daily reminders by the case manager and the attending, trainees recognize when information that must be entered in the medical record is time-sensitive, for example procedures or tests required for discharge. As my research progressed and case management no longer rounded with the IM team, the interns learned to self-regulate, taking turns staying behind to fill in the record as the team moved on to the next patient. As time went on and PMC shifted to 100 percent electronic record-keeping, interns learned to step away and take turns inputting information during morning rounds at computers centrally located throughout the wards, and then would promptly rejoin the team.

SPECIALISTS' IMPROPER USE OF THE MEDICAL RECORD

The medical record is a reminder to IM physicians of the need to routinely balance equally central yet often conflicting institutional logics at Pacific Medical Center. Learning how to properly use it is thus critical because of its potential to jeopardize the health, market, and legal logics and so disrupt patient care and generate both financial and legal consequences. However even if IM physicians learn how to properly use the medical record and ensure its proper use among team members, other parties may render it ineffective with improper documentation and use. This dilemma is particularly meaningful when IM physicians are dealing with consultants, who are routinely called at PMC. Intraprofessional work dynamics—particularly status hierarchies and associated assumptions of responsibilities for specific tasks such as notation—create conflicts when, from the perspective of the primary care team, specialists use the medical record improperly.

Improper use results when consulting teams see and treat IM patients but fail to provide notation, leaving IM physicians in the dark about clinical observations and treatment recommendations. In my interviews with both attendings and trainees, many said that Surgery and Transplant Services topped the list as the worst offenders. For instance, in a case involving a hypotensive, immunocompromised patient, IM physicians were frustrated with Renal Transplant's (RT) disregard of communication. The IM team was unable to continue treating the patient without having a discussion with RT first. An arterial blood gases test had been performed on the patient at five that morning. The resident knew that the RT team had administered the test; however, there was no notation as to who had administered it. Without knowing who treated the patient, the IM team had no information on the test results, which were integral to determining the patient's treatment options. The resident was visibly frustrated, muttering that she wished that RT "had just recorded it so we could know without having to contact them."

In a similar case, the IM team was at a standstill because of the lack of information about a male patient with a mass protruding from his head. During morning rounds, the resident explained that Neurosurgery had been concerned enough to order an emergent CT scan, which indicated that the mass should be drained. When the IM resident saw the patient earlier that day, there was a wrap on his head, but the resident was told that only Neurosurgery was allowed to examine under it. Unfortunately, there was no other information in the record about the procedure or the status of the mass. It was unclear to the team whether the mass had been drained and, if so, what it had been and how to proceed with care. Predictably, such communication failures often result in delays in care delivery and additional work for IM trainees, who must run down the missing information.

While the majority of dilemmas are caused by lack of notation, in a few instances consulting teams input orders directly into the patient's medical record without obtaining clearance from the primary care team, jeopardizing patient health and well-being. For example, Ms. Johnson, a middle-aged African American woman, had been transferred from Surgery to Internal Medicine after suffering a stroke during a routine splenectomy.[10] In preparation for the surgery, Ms. Johnson had been taken off of heparin, an anticlotting medication that was part of her daily care regimen. After several days on the IM wards, she had stabilized and was to undergo another surgical procedure. During morning rounds on the day of the procedure, Dr. Singh, the attending physician, grew very upset when Evelyn, one of the interns, notified him that the nurses had received orders from Surgery to once again take Ms. Johnson off her heparin because of the expected surgery. Dr. Singh angrily asked whether the intern had confirmed the order or had at least spoken with the surgical resident. The intern replied: "No, there were no orders or pages to me overnight." Evelyn said that the surgical resident had written the order without confirming the care plan with her. As a result, the nurses had merely followed orders and so Ms. Johnson was no longer on anticoagulation medication.

"She could have another stroke!" Dr. Singh shouted. He shook his head in disbelief, muttering that this was why she had been transferred to Internal Medicine in the first place. "*This* is why Surgery *should not* write orders." He directed Evelyn to have the surgical resident contact him immediately. He explained to the team that these situations were why the primary team *always* needs to write and implement orders, telling them that they needed to get input from Hematology (Hem) to determine the best course of action for Ms. Johnson since she still needed the surgical procedure but could not be taken off heparin.

Within the hour, the surgical resident had called and Dr. Singh asked the following questions: "Why was my intern not informed of the change in orders? Did you check with Hem about what to do? We *need* a recommendation from Hem in order to [figure out the] best course of action for this patient. She suffered a stroke because of the surgery preparation and this could have happened *again*." The call was brief. Later during rounds, the surgical resident, who had spoken with his own attending, told Dr. Singh that if the IM team did not want to be the primary team, Surgery would take Ms. Johnson back on their service. Visibly frustrated, Dr. Singh replied that they would remain Ms. Johnson's primary care team but would need full communication and discussion about her care plan.

The case of Ms. Johnson is a sobering reminder of how improper use of the medical record can endanger patients' lives. By failing to contact the primary care team and placing orders, Surgery not only left the team unaware of the patient's treatment plan but also placed her life at risk. While the most prominent concern of course was Ms. Johnson's health and well-being, adverse outcomes of such egregious medical errors could have left the physicians and the hospital particularly vulnerable to legal consequences.[11] The stakes for the IM attending, who was legally responsible for Ms. Johnson's care, were high. Unfortunately, notation conflicts are common—though mercifully not regularly associated with life-threatening health outcomes—amid the sharing of patients, reflecting professional dynamics and challenges that emerge in shared workplaces.

Shared-workplace dynamics inevitably shape perceived responsibilities and tasks related to patient care, directly blocking the objectives of the hospital's institutional logics. By actively documenting and using the medical record, trainees quickly recognize that the disregard of notation and its misuse reveal the implicit status hierarchies among physicians, where highly specialized physicians primarily focus on procedures and leave documentation and follow-up to the primary care team,[12] generating potential health, market, and legal ramifications for patients, physicians, and the hospital.[13] This topic will be explored in greater detail in the following chapter, but it is important to recognize how intraprofessional work dynamics deeply impact medical record documentation and consequently, patient care and outcomes.

DEFYING MARKET CONSIDERATIONS VIA THE MEDICAL RECORD

While the medical record reminds physicians of the importance of particular institutional logics when providing care, in some instances providers manipulate the medical record to prevent these logics from interfering in their care decisions. For instance, IM physicians often change the record in order to bypass the financial restrictions that guide the institution's market logic or to protect themselves and the hospital from litigation risks. Earlier I explored language-related disputes between insurers and providers via the medical record (a quick switch of a term resolves the problem) and dilemmas that arise when insurers challenge the medical decisions of the primary care team—often questioning whether a specific care decision is necessary and so eligible for coverage. Undoubtedly frustrating, such challenges come as no surprise to physicians, who have grown increasingly accustomed to third parties—especially insurers—contesting the decisions they make.[14] Insurer interference first became prominent in the 1970s, and by the 1990s, with the financial structuring of the health care system, insurer interference in medical decisions became common and expected.

Arguably, since the inception of medical insurance in the United States in the early twentieth century, interference in medical decision making was going to be inevitable. Initially, individuals received small-group health insurance through their employers or through mutual benefit associations such as fraternal organizations.[15] A pivotal change occurred in the late 1920s, when Baylor Hospital in Dallas, Texas, provided twenty-one days of hospitalization to its members for an annual payment of $6.00. Dallas teachers bought into this coverage, creating one of the first prepaid hospital insurance plans. Similarly, in 1929 Drs. Donald Ross and H. Clifford Loos created the Ross-Loos Medical Group, contracting with the Los Angeles Department of Water and Power to provide prepaid comprehensive health care to department employees and their dependents. This shift in how health insurance coverage was provided and to whom solidified two key components of coverage: first, insurance plans specifically designated to cover hospital care and, second, sickness insurance linked to one's work.[16]

The growth of the health insurance market accelerated during the Great Depression, which found both patients and hospitals in deep financial crisis. Hospitals' insufficient cash flow threatened their ability to remain open. In response, the American Hospital Association created prepaid hospitalization plans. These plans would guarantee cash flow to hospitals while lowering patients' financial responsibility for their care. One unforeseen consequence was competition among hospitals. To avoid competition, in 1939 Blue Cross was created as a network of hospital coverage plans. In 1946 Blue Shield was

established as a separate network for physician services.[17] In this early period, insurance plans were "pay as you go," where providers were guaranteed
payment—the primary goal of insurance plans at the time—and patients
did not pay any fees before their benefits kicked in. Plans thus covered all
medical costs without contention. In the mid-twentieth century, the health
insurance marketplace burgeoned with various plans and options: workplaces
increasingly offered employer-based health insurance and federal and state
governments became involved with the creation of Medicare and Medicaid
in 1965.

With various options accelerating during this time,[18] health care costs
began to rise exponentially. This was unsurprising considering that pay as
you go had no safeguards in place to limit health care spending; rather, the
primary objective was to protect provider and hospital compensation. Furthermore, neither patients nor providers were incentivized to reduce medical
care consumption: patients were fully protected from the costs of care so no
financial constraints factored into their decisions to seek care[19]; providers
were fully compensated for whatever care they delivered. In this way, the
structuring of plans and reimbursement in the first half of the twentieth century led to uncontrolled spending. In response, insurers adopted numerous
strategies, including increasing cost-sharing with patients—where patients
would take on more financial responsibility—and adopting managed care.[20]
In 1973 the Health Maintenance Organization Act propelled managed care,
creating federal agencies to facilitate development of HMOs.[21] The defining
characteristics of health maintenance organizations, which are in many ways
the hallmark of managed care,[22] include

> arrangements with selected providers to furnish a comprehensive set of
> health care services to members; explicit standards for the selection of
> health care providers; formal programs for ongoing quality assurance
> and utilization review; significant financial incentives for members to use
> providers and procedures associated with the plan.[23]

One of the key components of this care model was utilization management. Insurance companies assessed care decisions in the clinical setting
to "reduce excessive and unnecessary service utilization" and thus ensure
efficiency.[24]

To meet their utilization goals, managed care companies determined how physicians practiced medicine.[25] To the dismay of both patients and physicians, bureaucratic rules and practices quickly became entrenched in health care transactions.[26] Patients had a limited choice of medical practitioners and therapies, while physicians were limited in the patients they could see and the treatments they could provide.[27] Furthermore, limits were placed on how much time physicians could spend with patients,[28] resulting in increasingly shorter, more impersonal clinical encounters.[29] Also, insurers accepted or rejected care decisions, with rejection meaning no compensation to the provider, the patient, or both. Utilization review protocols were established to help control costs and theoretically improve care quality, the idea being that patients would avoid unnecessary care.

Nonetheless, high costs remain a serious concern, with both practice and policy changes specifically targeting care provision and insurance reimbursement policies. These changes bolster the influence of insurers in care decisions made in the clinical setting. At Pacific Medical Center, one of the most common financial conflicts between providers and insurers is over a patient's hospital stay; insurers often urge discharge before physicians feel a patient is ready. These assessments are made by a hired medical practitioner who simply reads through the patient's medical record, deciding that once a patient has been stabilized (according to the documentation), it is time for them to leave. The financial stakes of hospital discharge mean that it is highly scrutinized and contested by insurers. In response to pressures to cut costs and reduce medical waste, this push to quickly discharge patients has been a national initiative for several decades, and one can argue that it has been relatively successful. The 1999 National Hospital Discharge Survey reported that the average hospital stay in the US in 1980 was 7.3 days[30] versus in 2012, when the Health Care Cost and Utilization Project reported that the average hospital stay was 4.5 days.[31] Even with these modest improvements, however, safe patient discharge remains an ongoing challenge because of the complexities of hospital disposition.

Disputed discharges require IM physicians to reconcile their professional authority and autonomy with the restrictions placed on them in a highly commodified and bureaucratized health care system. They must weigh the costs and benefits for both patients and hospital. In this negotiation, physicians use the moral polysemy of the health logic to justify the decisions they make to meet different organizational objectives. Over the course of my research, it became clear that care decisions lacked uniformity aside from citing patient welfare as the determining factor. I saw many cases like Jordan's and Jessica's, where the IM physicians simply deferred to insurance restrictions. Yet there were as many cases where the IM team defied insurers and proceeded with a different care plan.

Although many decisions were made on a case-by-case basis, some commonalities emerged when IM physicians ignored insurers' demands. In such cases, they considered the gravity of the patient's condition, the likelihood that the patient would return to the hospital within a month or two, and litigation risk. If any of these factors raised a red flag, the IM physicians developed a care plan that contradicted the insurer's plan. IM attendings would teach trainees to proceed despite insurance restrictions by showing them how to alter a treatment plan or change the medical record. Minor changes always resolved any conflicts with insurers because they satisfied the insurer's checklist for "justified" treatments and hospital stays.

During my fieldwork, a common dispute between providers and insurers at Pacific Medical Center was the hospital stay. Physicians responded simply by altering the medical record to prolong a stay as needed, as one attending physician explained to me:

Let's say [the patient is] on oral Lasix. You put them on an IV Lasix dose and say we are diuresing the patient with [it]. That you can't do for an outpatient, so that will help you justify. Or if [the patient happens] to have a simple infection that would probably be okay to just put them on pill antibiotics, you just put them on IV antibiotics. Actually, we just admitted this patient overnight [who] had a pancreatic mass and [had gone] to an outside hospital to get the biopsy and to have a stent placed in their pancreas. The endoscopist there could not do the procedure—[the hospital was] not technically advanced enough—so they tried to get the patient transferred over to here. But the insurance company wouldn't cover it so they [discharged] the patient because they had nothing else to do. The patient had continued abdominal pain and came to our ER, and we were already hearing from the insurance company that he [needed] to be transferred elsewhere. So what [we did] in this situation was, because the patient had a fever two days ago, if the [the insurer] wanted to transfer him we [would tell them] he [was] unstable for transfer and just put him on IV antibiotics.

This story reveals how care decisions and treatment plans are modified simply for medical documentation. Physicians are highly skilled in convincing insurers to prolong a patient's hospital stay by switching therapeutic interventions from oral to intravenous.

I was told of an 87-year-old woman who had fallen in her home and fractured her arm. She required outpatient surgery yet remained in the hospital for pain control. Her family opposed a pending discharge because of her limited mobility and severe pain. The attending, Dr. Anand, agreed with the family and explained to the team during rounds that with arm fractures, typically, "there is not much of a mortality difference," so they tended not to keep the patient in the hospital. "They sometimes put a cast on it, reevaluate it, and then fix it. Sometimes they won't even fix it—especially if the patient is older and debilitated." In contrast, she continued, with hip fractures the patient always stays on the wards. Thus, to justify her stay to the insurance company, the medical record was altered to indicate that the patient's pain was being controlled by IV medications; this minor change kept the insurer at bay and revealed that age played an important role in the attending's determination to extend the length of stay. Elderly patients have greater potential for unexpected adverse health outcomes and immediate hospital readmissions, so they may be held longer while a younger patient with the same condition, such as an arm fracture, is discharged.

Dr. Anand recalled a time when she disagreed with an insurer's discharge decision. Her patient had cellulitis in his leg that was not improving, but the team's case manager had been notified that the insurer expected him to be discharged immediately. To Dr. Anand and her team, this decision was problematic and she was not comfortable discharging him with no monitoring of his condition. She told an intern to change the orders in the medical record to IV medication, which would ensure that the patient could stay in the hospital without insurer interference.

Such strategies illustrate a critical component of the medical record: what is written becomes the official—and only—documentation of care decisions and therapies administered. These decisions are shaped by numerous factors, including patient age, condition, support at home, and potential adverse outcome. Changes in notation are strategies to uphold the institution's health logic of ensuring patients' welfare with extended hospital stays. However, the legal logic features just as prominently in decision-making, if not more so, as adverse outcomes and allegations of medical negligence are key factors in medical litigation. Attending physicians frequently take into account that patients and families may claim medical negligence if they believe a poor health outcome was the result of being pushed out the door because of financial considerations.

Such clinical decisions can be juxtaposed with decisions to transfer patients like Jessica or Jordan out of the hospital: Why do Jessica and Jordan need to leave yet another patient can stay? Undoubtedly, the answer boils down to finances, primarily the patient's health insurance. I found that IM physicians were more comfortable editing medical documentation to extend patients' hospital stays if the patients were covered for care at Pacific Medical Center. Neither Jessica nor Jordan had coverage that would have allowed nonemergent care at PMC, leading their IM physicians to forgo strategies that would have extended their stay. Such examples once again reveal how a moral polysemy of the health logic invoked in discharge determinations causes inconsistent decision-making. Inconsistencies are frequently hidden by physician engagement with the health logic. The reality is that underneath the rhetoric of the health logic lie market and legal considerations that feature prominently in decision-making. The complex dynamics of hospital discharge will be explored in greater detail in Chapter 5, but it is important to note here that what is ultimately deemed the "best" for the patient is inevitably shaped by the patient's insurance, physicians' perceptions of patient resources and network, and their ensuing calculations of legal risk deriving from the decisions they make. Fear of litigation in medical practice and how it affects medical record use and documentation is explored next.

THE SIGNIFICANCE OF THE LEGAL LOGIC IN MEDICAL NOTATION

The fact that the medical record is a legal document that is read by numerous external parties leaves physicians vulnerable to legal recourse if any documented care decisions are deemed to be medically careless. At Pacific

Medical Center, IM physicians in particular are well aware of the significance of the medical record and the legal risk it entails. Attendings are in a unique situation, where they are legally responsible for care but are not primarily responsible for medical documentation. Thus, it is essential for them to convey to trainees the importance of meticulous notation and impress on them its professional stakes, which trainees are largely shielded from. Being meticulous can be confusing, however, because it can take on different meanings depending on the patient. Sometimes it requires that notes be comprehensive[32]; other times, it requires precise language and inclusion of only certain information. To dispel any ambiguity, many attendings micromanage notation, dictating to trainees exactly what should be written.

Micromanagement is particularly common when the legal stakes are high—for instance, when a proposed or prescribed treatment is not administered or a hospital stay is shortened at the request of the patient. In one case, a patient had been waiting for an MRI for several days. During this wait, his condition unexpectedly resolved, so the attending canceled the scan but ordered an intern to write in the patient's record "Condition had resolved itself before the study could be completed." He explained that this was necessary to justify the "failure" to complete the prescribed test.

As one might expect, documentation is particularly critical when there is a failure to follow recommended or prescribed treatment protocols. However, changes in care plans are not always made by physicians. In one example, against the recommendations of his primary care team a patient with stage four gastrointestinal cancer refused to undergo a PET scan at PMC, citing his limited financial resources. He remained steadfast even after numerous long conversations with his IM doctors. Upon leaving the patient's room, the attending directed an intern to precisely document (1) the physician's recommendation; (2) the patient's full capacity to make decisions; and (3) the patient's explicit refusal of the scan even after multiple discussions with his primary care team.

In another example, an attending physician was concerned about a patient's vegetative state and warned the team about carefully noting it in the medical record. During morning rounds, he explained that they may need to start thinking about how to approach the patient's family about her condition—she had been nonresponsive for five days—and directed an intern to place an order for a non-contrast MRI so that the team could look for evidence of altered mental status. Before the intern could begin the order, however, the attending interrupted: "You don't want to write 'evidence of a brain injury' but rather 'altered mental status' and/or 'the patient has been less responsive in the past few days.... You should always write 'less responsive,' not 'nonresponsive' . . . you don't want to *not* say something, but at the same time, you just need to be as nonspecific as possible. You never know, and hopefully won't ever be involved in a court case, [when] they tell you to turn to a particular page and it may be your notes. And then you need to explain why you wrote and did not write certain things in the order."

On occasion attendings directly edited trainees' notes if they flagged something as legally risky. Attending physicians' general management of medical notation stands in stark contrast to other aspects of care delivery, where trainees are given substantial license to make their own decisions and cultivate their own "doctoring" style in lab work requests, say, or bedside manner. I found that attendings were not always explicit with trainees about the potential risks of litigation, yet in interviews they raised concerns about them. One explained how medical documentation and fears of litigation can fuel certain care decisions: "The default in a place like this is often that more gets done so . . . someone [a consultant] will write a note and basically say it will be malpractice not to do X, [which] makes it hard for people not to do it." If the patient were to have a negative outcome and an investigation were performed, disregarding a documented recommendation could lead to severe professional and legal ramifications. Consequently, attending physicians readily acknowledge the significance of medical documentation and its implications for both patient care and the profession.

Unlike attendings, trainees have a very different perspective concerning the medical record and documentation. They expressed to me deep frustration over time-consuming medical notation, that it offered little pedagogical value. One third-year resident complained about the time spent writing "very complete notes where they document *everything.*"

Unsurprisingly, the practices and perceptions surrounding notation are directly shaped by level of training and position. As I mentioned earlier, trainees are sheltered from the legal responsibilities of patient care. The sentiments they expressed to me were not related just to notation; rather, some were surprised to see how much time was spent doing tasks like coordinating consultants and speaking with patients and families that seemed unrelated to clinical care.

Trainees' exasperation demonstrates the misalignment between professional expectations of what doctoring entails and the realities of inpatient work frequently encountered in clinical training.[33] Here it must be noted that one's specialty directly correlates with time spent on documentation. I observed that IM physicians at Pacific Medical Center spent more time on medical notation than specialists, which is a common phenomenon. A 2009 *Health Affairs* study found that primary care physicians everywhere spent more time than specialists and surgeons on administrative paperwork, especially that involving third party payers.[34] Realizing the sort of tasks that primarily filled their days,[35] some trainees opted to specialize as they progressed through their IM residency, although in my experience most stayed the course, and the unpopular tasks—including learning how to properly use the medical record—played a critical role in their professionalization, including the preemptive actions necessary to minimize the risk of litigation.

THE MEDICAL RECORD: CRITICAL LESSONS

The medical record is a vital document that is shaped by, and directly shapes, care delivery at Pacific Medical Center. How it is used—notation techniques and content—structures interactions among providers, patients, insurers, and relevant third parties. As trainees learn how to use the medical record, they also learn critical professional lessons about practicing medicine in the current health care system. In this way, the medical record plays an "active, constitutive role in current medical work . . . it is part and parcel of the production of hierarchical relations, of the shaping of the doctor-patient encounter, of the processes that constitute the socialization of interns."[36]

One of the critical lessons is how intraprofessional work dynamics on the clinical wards can disrupt the use of the medical record, jeopardizing the hospital's multiple institutional logics. Specifically, dependence on interspecialty care at PMC results in conflicts between IM physicians and specialists over documentation and the use and misuse of the medical record. Such conflicts cause delays and inefficiencies in care. Misuse, which is driven by a disregard for notation and effective communication with the primary care team, reminds trainees of how highly specialized medicine can be and the subsequent presence of intraprofessional status hierarchies, particularly at an elite academic institution like Pacific Medical Center. As their time on the wards progresses, IM trainees come to realize that disputes with specialists extend far beyond the medical record. In Chapter 4, I explore consultations at PMC, describing the challenges that trainees face and the critical lessons learned through the careful negotiation of patient sharing.

4 | CONSULTATIONS

Mrs. Park, a 40-year-old Korean American woman, came to the Emergency Department at Pacific Medical Center with meningitis, severe abdominal pain, and a rash. She was quickly assessed and admitted to the IM ward. Her primary care team asked Neurology to follow her. Mrs. Park was no stranger to the hospital: she had a history of recurrent meningitis infections that seemed to develop every two years. To the perplexity of her doctors, no one had been able to uncover their underlying cause. Upon evaluating Mrs. Park, Neurology recommended that the IM team consult Pain Management as well.

With three teams coordinating patient care, Mrs. Park stabilized within forty-eight hours. Her pain was better controlled after she received Dilaudid, a strong opioid, intravenously, but her rash remained. The IM team was unsure how to proceed and decided to ask Dermatology (Derm) to examine her. As the team convened during morning rounds on the third day of Mrs. Park's stay, a medical student reported that "there was no note left by Derm in the record after the consultant saw the patient," so he had been unable to move forward with a care plan.

"Oh. . . they called me and apologized for not leaving a note," the resident replied. "Derm felt this rash was not related to her meningitis and thought it could be rosacea. They recommended . . . steroids and to call back if they don't work." The medical student wrote down the plan and continued with his presentation. After some discussion, the team agreed that the primary goals were to get her out of bed and walking, and to approach her about discharge.

The following morning before rounds, Dr. Gehry, the attending physician, went to see Mrs. Park, in the hospital's Observation Unit. She was very drowsy and was holding an ice pack to her head. A nurse who was in the room told Dr. Gehry that Mrs. Park had been extremely upset that she had slept very poorly because she had not received the extra dose of pain medication she had requested. The doctor looked surprised as he assured the nurse and Mrs. Park that an order for an extra dose had been placed.

"Unfortunately, there was no documentation, so she was not given anything," the nurse said. Dr. Gehry apologized to the patient and her husband: "That is very strange. We will definitely fix the orders so she gets an extra dose . . . tonight, which she should have gotten last night as well."

As Dr. Gehry examined the patient, Mrs. Park and her husband raised additional concerns. There had been a change in her medications, and they were uncomfortable with this because Mrs. Park needed her previous medication. Mr. Park said that the new medication had "knocked her out for twelve hours straight," which they were both unhappy about. "I am here twelve to fifteen hours a day and for some reason Neurology has not been around to see us." Someone from Neurology was supposed to pay them a visit and give an update on the treatment plan and had not shown. Dr. Gehry agreed that this was unacceptable and said he would talk to the consultant. Mr. and Mrs. Park voiced dissatisfaction with the prescribed pain medication plan one more time, and Dr. Gehry promised to see what he could do. As we left the patient's room, Dr. Gehry told me: "The problem with the pain medication is that there are three teams covering this patient [Internal Medicine, Neurology, and Pain Management]. I am trained in Palliative Care and could play with the medication doses, but now with Pain Management onboard, we need to listen to them as well." He explained how much harder it was to appease three different teams as well as the patient when determining a treatment plan.

Before the end of her weeklong stay, Mrs. Park had four medical teams caring for her: Internal Medicine, Neurology, Pain Management, and

Dermatology. Her experience is a relatively routine one at PMC, where interspecialty care is both touted and expected given the hospital's mission and its complex patient population. However, sharing patients with consultants can create dilemmas and unexpected consequences. Ineffective communication was evident multiple times during Mrs. Park's hospital stay, leading to delays of necessary care and her increased discomfort. First, Dermatology failed to follow official communication protocols by not documenting its recommendation in the patient's record. This error might have been avoided had the consultant directly contacted the intern with care information, since typically interns (and in this case their medical students) are responsible for many daily care tasks. Because the resident was called, however, the intern and medical student were not privy to important treatment information until the team assembled during morning rounds. If the protocols had been followed, Mrs. Park's care plan could have moved forward more quickly. Instead, her rash remained unresolved. Also, although Mrs. Park was to receive additional pain medication overnight, there was no documentation of this order in her record so she went without and was in pain unnecessarily. She also had not approved changes that were made to her medication plan and was unable to speak to one of her specialists because they never visited her. Her primary care team, Internal Medicine, had assumed that care was proceeding as planned and only realized that things had gone wrong after she expressed her distress to the attending during morning rounds.

As discussed in Chapter 3, ineffective communication via the medical record is common, particularly when physicians share patients. Dr. Gehry admitted that part of the problem with Mrs. Park's pain care plan was bringing in Pain Management, although his training allowed him to manage pain, complicating communication and decision-making and raising the question: How was the health logic operating in this instance? Were consultants truly in the best interest of the patient? From a health perspective, as we see by the exchange between Mrs. and Mr. Park and Dr. Gehry, this was not the case. Dr. Gehry was frustrated, but he did not alter the plan.

When considering the primary intentions of the health logic, one could argue that it was not driving clinical decision-making in the case of Mrs. Park; rather, it was the financial and legal considerations that brought in and kept a consultant onboard. Dr. Gehry's frustration revealed his belief that

Pain Management was unnecessary, but his choice not to alter care points to a perceived lack of autonomy when making this choice. Arguably, IM physicians are not always making market and legal calculations when bringing in consultants, but these logics are embedded in the organizational culture at Pacific Medical Center, shaping health care professionals' assessments and decision-making such that it becomes a *given* that consultants will be called. Accordingly, IM physicians face both implicit and explicit pressures and expectations to provide interspecialty care that stem from PMC's multiple institutional logics.

It is important to note, however, that the challenges of interspecialty care are not solely due to contradictory institutional logics. The reliance on specialists is affected by the organization of the medical profession and intraprofessional work dynamics in the clinical setting. In Mrs. Park's case, the Dermatology consultant ignored the structuring of care delivery at PMC, where interns, primarily, coordinate daily care. In addition, these dynamics as well as intraprofessional status hierarchies shape how physicians across specialties approach various clinical tasks, including medical documentation. Ineffective communication and failure to properly document care decisions and protocols in the medical record result in delays of care, which have implications for both health and market logics.

First and most important, communication mishaps prolong a patient's distress. Second, delays of care can become costly if they compound over time and result in unnecessarily delayed discharge. Third, the work dynamics associated with patient sharing increase the likelihood of inefficiencies and ineffectiveness, with teams assuming too much or too little responsibility. Unfortunately, Mrs. Park's is not an exceptional case, but represents many of the challenges IM physicians face when they regularly count on specialists. This chapter explores how these physicians manage interspecialty care on the wards.

INTERSPECIALTY CARE AT PACIFIC MEDICAL CENTER

Sharing patients with numerous specialists is expected given the complex patient population routinely seen at academic medical centers like PMC. One attending physician explained:

We often don't see what's called "bread-and-butter medicine," very basic cases like pneumonia or just asthma. Usually, those patients can be triaged to another hospital—they don't necessarily need a bed *here*. So our patients either are complicated because they have had a transplant or they have been referred and transferred from another hospital because they require a higher level of care.

Dependence on interspecialty care is common in many US medical institutions and is largely driven by two factors: increased specialization and the fact that Internal Medicine is a generalist service.

One component of collaborative care at PMC is routine consultations to ensure quality, patient safety, and an amicable working environment. As discussed in Chapter 2, specialists have become a signifier of high-quality care, and having multiple specialists translates into more satisfied patients and improved health outcomes. At PMC consultations are deemed necessary to meet the objectives of the health logic.

Along with the health logic, consultants benefit the market and legal logics. The market logic sees specialists as associated with higher fees and care that is typically more complex and so profit-generating. They also serve the hospital's legal logic, as they may protect the primary care team and the hospital from litigation risk. When patients see that their care involves multiple specialties and greater expertise than offered by the IM team, fears of medical negligence may be assuaged. However, interspecialty care is rarely as straightforward as this. It becomes complicated because of contradictory institutional goals and objectives and intraprofessional work dynamics.

Social science scholarship on interdisciplinary work finds that its success is predicated on shared responsibility and decision-making[1] and mutual respect.[2] When there is a breakdown in any of these, teamwork becomes difficult. Different perspectives on responsibility and patient care commonly precipitate conflicts between the IM and consulting physicians at Pacific Medical Center. At the most fundamental level, the IM team is legally responsible for all patients on their wards: the attending is the physician of record. When disputes arise, the team has the final word. This rarely occurs, however, as intraprofessional work dynamics blur the boundaries when sharing patients.

The emergence and management of intraprofessional conflicts in the inpatient setting correspond with Abbott's seminal work on disputes between professional groups vying for jurisdiction over a specific arena.[3] Physicians are especially prone to jurisdictional disputes because they share knowledge, workplace, and even patients,[4] making disputes likely.[5] Ambiguous boundaries are particularly true of Internal Medicine and its subspecialties,[6] for which residents must first complete IM training. Interestingly, gastroenterologists train longer in Internal Medicine than in Gastroenterology in the United States.[7] Shared training further confuses jurisdictional claims. It generates questions about the expertise of one specialty over another and failure to recognize the need for collaboration.

Of particular significance are intraprofessional status distinctions and the hierarchical structuring of care delivery in teaching hospitals, exacerbating both ineffective communication and disputes between primary and consulting teams which have implications for patients and hospital alike. These include compromised patient care, unnecessary tests and procedures, costly delays of care, and extended hospital stays. IM physicians learn to manage status hierarchies to ensure smooth consultations. The remainder of this chapter explores interspecialty care, how it is disrupted, the strategies to manage its challenges, and its unintended consequences for physicians, their patients, and the hospital.

With interspecialty care frequently touted as optimal care that improves health outcomes and patients' experiences,[8] the Internal Medicine Service at PMC calls consults when they need help with a diagnosis or treatment plan, when a patient needs a procedure that only a specialist can perform, or when a patient's condition requires a specific specialty, such as Renal Transplantation.[9] At Pacific Medical Center, the atmosphere surrounding consultations is palpable, with internists feeling pressured to call consultants and consultants feeling pressured to provide a recommendation for a test, procedure, or treatment protocol. In seamless consultations, consultants readily agree to assess the patient and provide timely, straightforward recommendations[10] that the IM team accepts and proceeds with accordingly. Tests or procedures are completed with minimal interaction across services other than the pages, notes, and phone calls necessary to coordinate care. Collaborations are smooth, and there is little disagreement over treatments. However, consultation is complicated by the hospital's training logic and the hierarchical structuring of care delivery based on level of training.

As mentioned, IM trainees monitor and coordinate the bulk of patient care. Interns generally initiate all contact with specialists, who are either fellows or attending physicians, but they have minimal interaction with them in non-teaching settings.[11] This difference in status and experience between the IM team and the consultant can lead to problems. For instance, interns may request a consult and the specialist may refuse, or block, the request, which can negatively affect patient health and well-being if specialty expertise is needed.

Blocking can be attributed to variations in clinical experience and to professional status hierarchies. First, inexperienced trainees may provide insufficient information when initiating a consult, leaving specialists questioning whether they are truly needed. During one monthly IM hospitalist meeting, a gastroenterologist (GI) said that consultations could be improved with better education of IM interns, who occasionally called the GI fellow about a patient whom they had never actually seen. This became problematic when the fellow requested mandatory information such as the patient's name, the patient's location, and the time sensitivity of the patient's condition (thirty minutes, one hour, etc.). If an intern had not seen the patient, these questions were unanswerable.

To avoid such issues, contacting consultants with a precise question or set of questions is key. Housestaff must learn to gather sufficient information on the patient before making a consultation request. A second-year resident in Emergency Medicine spoke to me about properly initiating a consult:

> [In the second year] in Emergency Medicine, you're more aware of what a consultant needs to have or needs to know about the patient *before* we call them. In your intern year, you tend to call consultants before you actually have your question formulated so that the consultant can answer [it], and sometimes you actually call the consultant before workup has been completed. But in your second year, you realize that if you're calling an orthopedic surgeon, you have to wait for your imaging, even if the patient clinically has an orthopedic need. Or if you're calling a urologist, you have

to wait for imaging and labs, such as a urinalysis, to make sure that you have all the information needed to formulate the question you want to ask.

Unsurprisingly, attending physicians are the ones who teach trainees how to ask the right questions. One day during morning rounds, the IM team was discussing an elderly patient. They were unsure how to proceed because they were awaiting the results of her TEE (transesophageal echocardiography).[12] She had fluid overload, and the one thing the team knew was that they needed to remove some of the fluid. The attending told the team that if the patient did not improve soon, they would need to broaden her treatment plan. The resident agreed and proposed calling the Pulmonary fellow. The attending then said, "We may have reached a point where we need to read more and ask a specialist about her condition." He then identified the key issues and the questions that the intern should ask the pulmonologist. First, "[The patient] continues to have a high oxygen requirement, and we tried diuresing her but she is not getting better, so what do we do?" Second, "[The patient] has two infections that must be considered. She is on Vanco for one of them. We are not treating the second yet because the TEE results are unavailable as yet. Should we be considering putting her on Colistin?" Third, "Is it worthwhile for us to insert a chest tube for her pleural effusion? Though probably a TEE is better and more appropriate than a chest tube." And fourth, "Is a CT a good idea?" An intern jotted down the questions and the team wrapped up their discussion armed with a much clearer treatment plan.

On another occasion, an attending physician stopped an intern from prematurely calling a consultant with insufficient information. An 83-year-old man who had recently undergone a thirty-five–pound weight loss, had been admitted to PMC with generalized weakness and malnourishment. After a CT scan, the team found possible metastatic disease. The patient had a large mass on his spleen, but his prostate-specific antigen was normal, which was confounding. As a result, a biopsy was performed. During morning rounds, the intern told the attending that he planned to consult Hematology-Oncology (Hem-Onc) to address the patient's potential metastatic disease. "Let's see what the biopsy shows," the attending suggested. "Splenic mets[13] of that size are uncommon." The resident agreed: "Let's first see if the colonic mass is there, to save money on unnecessary workup. It's weird for it to be cystic."

A few days later, the patient was scheduled for a PET[14] scan. Once again at morning rounds, the intern asked if he should contact Hem-Onc. The attending stated that they should wait for the scan because their questions would change based on its results. The intern nodded and reviewed the plan. "Okay. So wait and see if there is anything biopsy-able from the PET scan, and then call Hem-Onc if that is the case. If there is nothing, call Hem-Onc the next day to discuss anticoagulation for the patient once discharged."

Blocking may result not only because interns fail to provide appropriate information at the outset but also because of the hierarchical nature of medicine. IM physicians at Pacific Medical Center immediately encounter intraprofessional hierarchies of skill and expertise when they begin to practice on the wards. One hierarchy is revealed by specialists who are unlikely to be convinced by an intern to follow a patient. The status distinction between the intern and the consultant can shape consultations and patient care across medical teams; interns in particular may find it difficult to challenge specialists.[15] They may try to cajole: "My attending *really* wants you to take a look at this patient" and be met with variable success. Numerous IM attendings expressed frustration with how their interns were treated by consultants. In a brief conversation with me after rounds, one angrily stated, "And [for] other services, you have to sit down for twenty minutes with the intern to coach them on exactly what to say or else basically the consulting fellow is going to try to block the consult and be downright condescending and abusive, almost hostile, toward your intern. . . . I've had some *very* bad experiences recently with consult services."

An important reminder is that consulting fellows are themselves trainees and find themselves buried by work because of the structuring of care delivery in teaching institutions. They may refuse to take on a case to minimize their workload. Financial disincentives may also discourage some consultants from taking on patients. An attending physician discussed with me the financial barriers to successful consultations:

> Consultants from surgical subspecialties are asked to cover for many different services. There are few [surgical] housestaff for many patients and many consultations. So they generally do not [come] by as much. The attendings often do not come in to see those patients unless they are going

to go operate. And at that point, they only see them in the operating room. They only do that because they get paid to operate, not to consult. Their time is better spent in the OR. They don't bill for the consultation whereas in the Department of Medicine, they do. So the [surgeons] have a financial disincentive to do things unless there is an indication for a procedure. You have less input and sometimes you have to prod them more to do things.

Unfortunately, then, even with the right information and questions, the IM team can be met with refusal.

When a consultant refuses to see an IM patient, the IM attending directly contacts the consulting fellow or attending, bypassing the bottom-up approach typical of academic medical centers. The attending may provide details about the patient's condition that were not in the initial request. Or the team may "massage" the presentation of medical evidence in order to persuade a reluctant specialist, such as with tests revealing compelling medical data or altered care plans.

In one case, a Gynecology consultant blocked a request for an inpatient consult. The IM attending believed that the patient needed to remain in the hospital because of her pain. Discussing the patient during morning rounds, he urged the team to be careful when administering pain medications; he did not want her pain to go away too quickly, reasoning that if it did, the consultant would dismiss the patient, convinced that she should be discharged. The primary goal of this strategy was to demonstrate that the consultant's expertise was crucial to the patient's care. Such strategies are usually successful, but they highlight an important fact: like interns, IM attending physicians encounter challenges to care delivery due to intraprofessional status hierarchies.

Increasing stratification based on specialization places generalists at the bottom of the status totem pole.[16] Thus, in some instances IM attendings are expected to defer to novice consulting physicians simply because of their specialization. According to Dr. Gehry,

Unfortunately, I have seen some—mostly minor—issues result: maybe longer length of stay, higher expense of health care, unnecessary tests, anxiety, procedures. I see that happen a little bit less with more experienced consultants, but we have a fair turnover here of people that are right out of their fellowship. . . . You will get into some strange situations where since this is my *tenth* year practicing here now, I may have a fellow that's been practicing all together for six years or so. And I may have possibly even seen more cases of something that falls within their specialty, and they want me to do one thing, and I want to trust them and respect their opinion, but I may feel strongly that we should do something else.

These comments reveal how status hierarchies create disagreement in regard to treatment trajectories and support resolutions that can negatively impact the patient's physical or emotional health, as well as lead to unnecessary inpatient spending.

The inability to refuse a specialist's recommendation is most viscerally experienced by trainees. As one might expect, interns are deeply uncomfortable questioning consultants' recommendations and so immediately execute their orders for diagnostic procedures and treatment plans without always conferring with their own attendings or even pausing to consider whether such orders are truly necessary or in the best interest of the patient. This is especially true in the Emergency Department and overnight, when residents must manage patients on their own. In some cases, even before the patient has been officially admitted to the Internal Medicine Service or has been seen by the attending physician, numerous consultants will already be onboard. One attending spoke wearily about the organization of care delivery at Pacific Medical Center:

You know, if you work in a hospital with residents—where the residents call all of these consultants—sometimes the consultants get called *before* you even see the patient yourself. So, in the emergency room there is a person with a lung problem and the lung doctors have already come around and they say what they think, or there is a person with a rash and the dermatologist has come by, or there is a person with a swollen knee and the rheumatologist has come by, and so sometimes you don't have control over whether the consultants come around.

Status hierarchies generate problematic consultations, as the expectation of deference to superiors not only can lead to excessive care but can have little impact, or a negative one, on a patient's health and well-being.

Once during postcall rounds,[17] the resident on the IM team recounted a traumatic overnight event that involved one of their newly admitted patients. She explained that the patient did not want vancomycin because he was allergic to it. The consultant, however, argued that the patient needed the drug. "We didn't know what to do. Ultimately, we gave the patient vancomycin because when the consultant is the chair of Lung Transplant, what *can* you do?" She explained that the patient went into anaphylactic shock and was immediately intubated. Fortunately, he was doing fine now. The attending's silence spoke volumes, affirming that in this situation little could have been done: an IM resident is powerless when the consultant is the chair of a specialty service. This is a perfect example of how the structuring of care delivery at teaching hospitals, and the intraprofessional work dynamics that emerge through patient sharing, complicate the consultation process, in some instances greatly compromising the hospital's health logic by endangering patients' lives.

A CULTURE OF COLLEGIALITY: ACCEPTING THE ROLE
OF CONSULTATIONS IN CARE DELIVERY

At their best, consultations vastly improve patients' experiences and health outcomes but they can also lead to unnecessary costs that negatively affect the market logic. Often thought of as profit generating, consultations mean more care. More care is not problematic if it is necessary; however, at PMC and hospitals across the country, frequently "more is not better." Interspecialty care increases the likelihood that patients will receive care that is not needed and that frequently prolongs their hospital stay. The financial costs of interspecialty care are increasingly discussed by health care professionals with concerns that, because it is the current system default, it drives spending without improving health outcomes.[18] At Pacific Medical Center, IM physicians share these concerns, with many often questioning the necessity of a treatment or test. The majority of physicians are frustrated with PMC's orientation toward consultations, displeased with their overuse and questionable effectiveness. In a conversation about the consequences of calling consultants, one attending said,

> There are some consult teams that you are hesitant to unleash. I won't name any specific teams, but you say, "Oh shoot! Do we have to consult

such and such a team?" Because the minute we do, we are going to have to send off thirty-eight laboratory tests or start different medications that may not necessarily be indicated quite yet. There are strong personalities on different consult teams and they may have a different view from a generalist which is, you know, "less is more" sometimes,—I have seen [inappropriate] tests sent off. And once you find one little abnormality on one test, you go to the next test and then the more invasive test and the more invasive test past that.

Overtreatment and overuse of medical resources are common consequences of interspecialty care. Such was the case when a 27-year-old man, admitted to the Internal Medicine Service at PMC with recurrent gastrointestinal bleeding, was being followed by Gastroenterology and Vascular Surgery. As the patient stabilized, his discharge was pending. During morning rounds, the resident on the primary care team I was following questioned the need for a specific therapy recommended by the gastroenterologist. The attending dismissed the plan and explained to the team: "Calling consultants . . . it's sort of like hot potato: 'You're it!' And now what do you do?" This implicit pressure to "do something" when consulted often leads to unnecessary care. In an interview, a first-year intern said, "When you're called as a consult, you're *expected* to provide recommendations. And the recommendation is never not to do anything or to do less. It's always 'do these tests, do this, do that.' They're kind of expected to give you things to do if you're going to call them."

An attending mentioned that he frequently encountered specialists whose approach to care directly contradicted the generalist's "less is more":

A lot of surgical services have [IM] doctors comanage their patients for their medical problems. This whole management model is really growing—I think it started with Orthopedic Surgery and Neurosurgery. Whenever they admit patients to their services, they also want Internal Medicine onboard to follow the patient throughout the whole hospital stay—address all the other issues. But then . . . different surgeons have different thresholds for calling consultants. If there's a little problem with the heart, they call cardiologists. People spike a fever; they call infection doctors. There's some issue with sugars, and they call diabetes doctors.

So it's not uncommon that, somewhere along the path, we have a lot of different doctors involved and a lot of times it's *really* unnecessary and excessive.

This observation emphasizes that many consultation disagreements are a consequence of specialization. As physicians increasingly specialize, fundamental differences arise in how they are trained to think about, and approach, different health concerns. They attribute "different weights to the same sickness situations, according to the perspectives and approaches that characterize each of the skills."[19] I heard an attending express both gratitude and relief that his team had surprisingly fewer consultants onboard than normal: "Enjoy the unusual experience of no aggressive consultants making demands on us."

The obvious solution would be for the IM team to simply reject recommendations they deem unnecessary. Doing so can be rather difficult, however, because, similar to the pressure to routinely call consultants, there is institutional pressure to *accept* all recommendations. Many IM physicians explained that there is a "culture of collegiality" at PMC that drives the expectation that specialists' recommendations will not be contested, so questioning them or rejecting care plans often becomes synonymous with burnt bridges and frosty relationships. Because the inpatient setting requires frequent and repeated collaboration with colleagues, they are careful to preserve good relationships with them. One attending explained that, if her team called a consult and the consultant recommended an additional service, she accepted this recommendation even if she did not want to. She would rather "keep it collegial." Another attending had felt the same way:

> If the primary team and the consulting team disagree, it's ultimately the primary team's decision. . . . However, you also have to take into account that most of us work in the same hospital. If I consult Pulmonary, and they want to do a bronchoscopy and I disagree, I often say okay to the bronchoscopy because I don't want to anger my pulmonologist. I know that I'm going to have to consult them tomorrow or next week, right? So there is some congeniality. If it's a small thing or your goals are pretty close . . . then you often go with what the consultant says even if you don't think it's necessary.

Dr. Gehry described a patient case he had been consulted on where his clinical judgment was superseded by another specialist's recommendation, resulting in a chain reaction of unnecessary consults, tests, and procedures:

I was following a patient postoperatively who had a history of lupus nephritis—kidney damage due to lupus. And I followed her closely for about six or seven days. Her creatinine—the monitor of her kidney function—had slightly decreased a few days after surgery. I was [almost a hundred percent] convinced that she *just* needed more fluid. They needed to give her a couple liters of fluid through the IV and her problems would be solved. I was a consultant on the case myself. And then the OB-GYN team, the main team taking care of the patient, called the Rheumatology team, who hadn't been following the patient for the six days that we had. It's really hard to tease out everything that happened in that time period. When you're a hammer, the world looks like a nail, so they ordered all sorts of testing. They told the team to get another consult—a nephrology consult—which I didn't think was indicated. And they ordered things like a renal ultrasound and many other lab tests to see if lupus was actively injuring the kidney.

I think all [the patient] needed was a two-dollar bag of saline and her problem would have been solved. But you know, like I said, when you're a hammer. . . . It's very tough as a consultant to get called about something that's in your specialty and not do anything about it. It takes a very experienced consultant to say, "You don't need any test. This clearly isn't lupus nephritis. Leave the patient alone and give them some fluid like the medical consultant said, and let's save us all a lot of time and money."

Experiences like Dr. Gehry's are common at Pacific Medical Center. Collegiality preserves good relationships across services that are routinely expected to work together as required for quality inpatient care in the long run. IM physicians frequently calculate the costs and benefits of interspecialty care and always try to follow PMC's cultural approach: they rely on it heavily, even if they perceive that specialist involvement may not dramatically improve a patient's condition.

Consultation emerges as yet another interesting site of moral polysemy in care delivery. While seemingly operating according to the health logic when working with consultants, physicians are actually motivated to share patients by organizational, professional, and legal pressures. Yet unlike clinical decisions, such as discharge determinations, which can vastly differ across patient cases, generally the outcome of consultations is uniform: the consultant is called and the recommendation is accepted. Here we see a slightly different form of moral polysemy than the one that Altomonte discusses: although physicians draw on organizational and legal considerations when making decisions, the outcomes themselves are rarely divergent. Arguably, consultations are where organizational and professional needs and culture align so strongly that IM physicians have less agency than when making other care decisions and there is less room for alternative options. Still, the IM team continues to share patients with specialists regardless of the implications for patient health and well-being.

While the organizational culture around consultation would appear to mitigate disputes, the following section examines how conflicts cannot always be avoided. To prevent negative ramifications for both patient and hospital, IM physicians must learn to diffuse problematic situations that inevitably arise in routine collaboration on the wards.

WHOSE PATIENT? CONFLICTS THROUGH COLLABORATION

The most common dispute between the IM and consultant teams during my fieldwork was the overstepping of jurisdictions—that is, when a single team (IM or consulting) sought complete ownership of patient care and failed to collaborate with the others. In many of these conflicts, consulting teams did not adequately communicate with the primary team or refused to compromise when coordinating patient care to reach a single treatment plan. Such dynamics arise when certain physicians are granted greater status than others.[20] Some doctors higher-placed in the hierarchy may ignore "nonprofessional issues or irrelevant professional issues from practice"[21] and consequently dismiss tasks they consider mundane, like long conversations with patients and family members.[22] Others may ignore the concerns of their colleagues or refuse patients with conditions perceived as tedious.[23] The desire to only practice specific skills shapes how specialists and generalists approach patient care and each other, resulting in conflicts that reinforce divisions and increase the likelihood of exclusion of particular groups from decision-making.[24]

Dr. Gehry discussed the difficulties encountered when several teams try to dictate patient care rather than collaborate:

> I remember a consultation on a patient who was admitted with some finger swelling, which suggested a rheumatologic condition, but it was pretty vague and, in my opinion, was relatively benign. I don't think it was something that warranted an acute hospital stay necessarily. But the referring physician was a subspecialist and had then done the consultation. [The subspecialist] asked for at least three or four separate consultations from Vascular Surgery, Gastroenterology, and Hematology—involving a series of things that were excessive in my opinion. . . . That certainly led to some conflict over what to do because particularly housestaff, who are more junior . . . are caught between the primary attending and the consultant, who is trying to drive the course of management. Instead of a collaborative approach, sometimes you have a situation where they're telling the house officers what to do, and the house officers feel obliged to do it since the consultant is more senior.

In another conversation, a second-year resident described how difficult it could be to convince specialists to collaborate effectively, noting services that regularly contradicted one another: "There are certain consult teams that tend to fight each other. . . . So having Cardiology and Renal onboard at the same time *always* means that you're going to have conflicting recommendations. Same with Hem-Onc and Rheumatology."

Often in such cases, the role of Internal Medicine as the "primary" medical team ultimately in charge of patient care, is often overlooked. How do IM physicians respond? Similar to disputes over the medical record, when specialists ignore shared jurisdiction, the IM team uses the hierarchical structuring of medicine to their advantage: they explicitly move up the medical hierarchy to prevent or deescalate conflicts. In these cases, the training logic at Pacific Medical Center is ignored and the care delivery model is inverted. In routine consultations, housestaff from the IM team and fellows from the consulting team correspond throughout the patient's stay. In contrast, conflicts due to opposing recommendations from various consulting services are reconciled by the IM team's *bypassing* of negotiations between housestaff and fellows, with IM attendings directly contacting the attending consultants—excluding trainees from the process. Inversion diffuses unwanted interactions generated by the hierarchy of the medical profession and medical training in teaching hospitals.

All of the trainees and attending physicians I spoke to said that, when disagreements arose, the IM attending acted as an intermediary—bridging divergent opinions until a single treatment plan was reached. The attending either spoke to each consultant individually or coordinated a meeting with all consultant attendings involved in patient care. While not all meetings went smoothly or quickly, IM attending involvement signaled to specialists that resolution would be necessary. Consultants would have to agree on the importance of directly contacting attendings in certain cases. This strategy established an interdependent division of labor among physicians in which specialty services' recommendations were combined to create one comprehensive treatment plan. The crucial role of communication is supported by the clinical scholarship: the way to manage and prevent conflicts among consultants is to improve the flow of information through the use of communication guidelines.[25]

To this point, the examples here have focused on the failure of consulting teams to share jurisdiction. However, IM physicians, too, can refuse to share. One key factor in this is that trainees want to advance their training and education and thus want a first shot at patient management before seeking help from a specialist. During an Internal Medicine Service monthly hospitalist meeting I observed,[26] gastroenterologists complained that IM physicians were too hesitant to consult their service. They explained that morbidity and mortality from gastrointestinal conditions were primarily due to slow communication in acute cases. The most common and critical problem was the tendency to treat a patient with a gastrointestinal bleed as a *medical* case rather than a *surgical* one; if the patient was losing blood, the gastroenterologists said, there was no time to waste.

Endocrinologists had similar complaints with IM physicians. One endocrinologist presented a case that revealed the deadly consequence of hesitating to call Endocrinology. A patient with hypopituitarism had been admitted and received prednisone (steroid) treatment. His condition worsened and he required intubation. While being intubated, the patient went into cardiac arrest. He was transferred to the Intensive Care Unit, where he eventually died.

The Endocrine consultant was contacted *after* the arrest, but the patient had been in the hospital for six days prior to the consultation and the Endocrine team felt that had it been consulted earlier perhaps the patient's death could have been averted. This case was a sobering lesson for IM physicians: failing to share jurisdictions can become a matter of life or death.

The IM physicians acknowledged that their trainees were sometimes inappropriately hesitant to call consultants, and they provided anecdotes: an IM resident failed to consult Rheumatology for a patient admitted to the service after falling at home. The patient received an x-ray and lay in bed unable to move for several days. Once Rheumatology was called, and within two days, the patient was mobile again. The delay in calling Rheumatology prolonged the patient's discomfort and his hospital stay. After conversations with specialists like the ones just described, the IM attendings agreed to better educate their trainees to initiate consults quickly and, when uncertain if a consult was necessary, always err toward interspecialty care.

A professional factor that may exacerbate hesitation is the overlap of medical knowledge across specialties that leads to different opinions on who should ultimately have jurisdiction over a condition or procedure.[27] For instance, during a meeting between Internal Medicine and Endocrinology, the endocrinologists asked to be consulted on all cases of hyponatremia, a metabolic condition characterized by insufficient sodium in body fluids. The IM physicians disagreed: Internal Medicine was often consulted by *other* specialty services, such as Neurology, to manage their hyponatremia patients. The endocrinologists also said that, because insulin management was specific to their specialty, they should be consulted on it. The IM physicians disagreed once again, arguing that insulin management fell within the purview of internists. As these vignettes show, similar training experiences can confuse who should be responsible for certain conditions, resulting in IM physicians, particularly housestaff, being hesitant to contact consultants. They also reveal how an orientation toward consultations can directly compromise the hospital's health and legal logics, as adverse outcomes come at great cost to patient health and well-being and leave physicians and the hospital vulnerable to legal recourse.

It is not surprising that differences in perspective on interspecialty care frequently fall along training lines. Echoing comments made during interspecialty meetings, in their interviews attendings raised concerns that trainees were sometimes too cavalier in their approaches to care. In their interviews, trainees frequently labeled attendings too conservative. Many believed that attendings relied on specialists too much and, because of the culture of defensive medicine, routinely requested unnecessary consultations that could be handled by Internal Medicine. As one second-year resident explained,

> There are a lot of times that the attending wants me to consult but I feel like we don't need to. It's something that *we* should be able to handle as Internal Medicine doctors on our own. . . . But . . . I can understand it from the attending's perspective because they're ultimately the physician of record. . . . A lot of times we call consults as a sort of "cover your ass" thing. It's a situation where *you* know what the right thing to do is but you think an "expert" should be onboard to back you up. So I can understand it from that perspective because I'm not ultimately the one who is liable.

Although acknowledging the fear of litigation, many trainees begrudged the institution's legal logic and the tendency of attendings to practice defensive medicine, which the trainees perceived as inhibiting their learning and "true medical work."

From the trainees' perspective, consultations bogged them down with duties that did little to advance their medical knowledge. Consultations often led to more work but fewer opportunities to test their skill, gain confidence in their abilities, and prove themselves as novice physicians. The trainees agreed that it was easy for attendings to request a consultation since trainees were the ones who had to actually correspond with specialists and coordinate patient care. Medical training leaves housestaff burdened with heavy workloads that disincentivize calling consultants.[28] When faced with seemingly unnecessary consults, trainees would contact the fellow and preface the request with "I'm sorry to do this but my attending is asking for a consult."

Collectively, the examples in this chapter show that the training logic places interns at the forefront of consultations—where they must balance status hierarchies against their desire to advance their clinical knowledge. Furthermore, specialty services do not necessarily duck responsibilities or disregard the institution's health logic, but with their different approaches to clinical knowledge they directly influence approaches to patient care.

THE STAKES OF CONSULTATIONS

Patient well-being, inpatient spending, and legal risk are all aspects of hospital care that are influenced by how collaborative care is managed. Ineffective consultations have the potential for poor health outcomes, leaving both physicians and the hospital vulnerable to claims of medical malpractice. Consultations can also become costly if they create medical waste, delays of care, and in turn discharge delays. Specialists approach care in contradictory ways, which leads not only to divergent treatment plans but also to divergent discharge plans. Many of the IM physicians I interviewed expressed irritation that consultants often complicated a pending discharge. One intern described a common occurrence in patient sharing: "We might be trying to get a patient out . . . but the consult team is not on the same page and says, 'Oh [the patient] can stay as long as we need.'" IM physicians try to prevent discharge delays by agreeing with consultants on a single care plan before talking with the patient and family, but this is not always possible or successful.

Another factor that shapes the reliance on consultations is the patient. As patient satisfaction has become central to health care initiatives and institutions, patients have become emboldened to take their rightful place at the decision-making table. They are growing more comfortable demanding more care, more consultants, and more interventions. Health care professionals are likely to bend to these requests, especially when they fear legal recourse. In particular, patients' voices are increasingly vocal in discharge planning at Pacific Medical Center, often pushing for extended stays. The following chapter explores hospital discharge in depth: what successful discharge management entails and how physicians learn to navigate the contradictory objectives of the hospital's multiple institutional logics in discharge determinations.

5 | DISCHARGE

Ms. Farhad, a 90-year-old woman of Middle Eastern descent with advanced gastric cancer, was admitted to the Internal Medicine Service at Pacific Medical Center after experiencing vomiting and weakness for four weeks, and had been at another hospital one week prior to her PMC admission. She was hypotensive when she was assessed in the Emergency Department, where she remained while awaiting an open bed on the IM wards. Once the IM team had assembled at a computer station, Michael, the medical student assigned to Ms. Farhad, began his presentation by reviewing the patient's medical history, labs, and vitals. Amina, the resident, who was quickly looking over the patient's chart, interrupted: "Her bicarb [has] dropped significantly."

"Has her renal function gotten worse?" Dr. Brandon, the attending physician, asked.

"It's better now," Michael replied.

"Yes, her renal function is improving but her bicarb has dropped," Amina repeated.

"Is the patient full code?" asked Dr. Brandon.

"Right *now* she is full code because we are unaware." Amina responded. "But we must talk to the family to find out whether she is or not."

Dr. Brandon sighed. "Ok, let's wait and talk to them . . . before we do anything aggressive."

Michael listed his treatment recommendations for Ms. Farhad: "I would like to consult Surgery and GI [Gastroenterology], primarily because the patient's G-tube seems to be leaking feces."

"That's weird, right?" Amina interjected. "The patient hasn't been eating or drinking though."

"Definitely feces?" Dr. Brandon asked.

Amina nodded. "Yes, it is very foul smelling." She then turned to Michael and told him to page Gastroenterology. Michael immediately input the page and reiterated that he would clarify the patient's code status. After some consideration, Amina stated, "For now, I am ok with *just* a GI consult."

"But what about consulting Surgery?" Michael questioned.

Amina shook her head, "No, they will say she has no obstruction and dismiss [her]."

On the way to see Ms. Farhad, Amina received a call from the Gastroenterology fellow. "Wow, that was quick!" Dr. Brandon exclaimed.

In the Emergency Department, Amina spoke in Farsi with the family members and translated for the team. They had a brief conversation about the patient's symptoms and the family's preference not to escalate care. As the team members filed out of Ms. Farhad's room, Amina remarked, "I know in my culture they try to solve it all [medically], so it can be a painful conversation but fortunately not this time." In response to the goals-of-care conversation, Michael called Palliative Care.

The first twenty-four hours with Ms. Farhad represented a critical lesson for trainees: establishing goals of care with the family upon patient admission. It is crucial to determine *how* the family wants to approach care as early as possible to ensure a plan that is approved by all parties. Dr. Brandon's request for the patient's code status is an essential one, reminding trainees that this information directly impacts the treatment decisions the IM team will make. Why does this matter? Effective communication with the family helps the team determine a patient's care trajectory, including a discharge plan, that aligns with the patient's and family's wishes. This approach promotes inclusion of patient and families in care decision-making (which builds patient satisfaction and deflects accusations of medical negligence), avoids unnecessary medical care and discharge delay (because the patient and family and the IM team are on the same page), and keeps the primary care team aware of potential barriers to discharge that may stem from patient or family concerns. Effective communication sets up a successful discharge plan that aligns with the institution's health, market and legal logics.

By day two of Ms. Farhad's hospital stay, the gastroenterologist had seen her and was confident that there was no obstruction in her G-tube. Much of the patient's condition remained unchanged, and her family had rejected a repeat computed tomography (CT) scan that had been ordered overnight.

"What are the ultimate goals of care? How aggressively do we want to treat this patient?" Dr. Brandon asked the team during morning rounds.

"I talked to the family again yesterday and I feel it is not safe for her to go home without hospice," Amina responded and then brought up a potential issue with the family: Palliative Care had left a note in Ms. Farhad's record stating that the family did not want the patient to go home with hospice but did not want to escalate care either.

"I think," said Dr. Brandon, that "we need to think about the long term since she's not going to die imminently. A couple of lab tests or a cortisol injection would be fine, but bigger tests and treatments. . . . I'm not sure whether [we should] do procedures like an echo [echocardiogram] . . . so a good start would be to talk to the family again and figure out where they stand." As the team agreed, Amina noted that Ms. Farhad was also hypotensive and she did not know why.

"Is she on opiates?" Dr. Brandon asked. Michael told him she was not. Because pain seemed not to be a major feature, Dr. Brandon suggested "some enemas or suppositories . . . and we could try and decompress her from below."

"I *still* don't know what we are treating yet," Amina sighed in frustration. Dr. Brandon nodded sympathetically as he replied: "The family seems reasonable at least." Amina agreed although she remained concerned of their hesitation regarding hospice, which was needed for this patient. She muttered, "It seems they *would consider* hospice because they would like to do nothing—no invasive care." Dr. Brandon suggested that the family was "probably resistant to a nursing home for cultural reasons."

Amina's grappling with the tension between her assessment that the patient needed hospice and the family's resistance to it was another teachable moment for the trainees: proper care and discharge management require not just early but *consistent* conversations with the family—not a single conversation at the start of the patient's stay and another one about a discharge plan but rather an ongoing dialogue to account for the wishes of the patient and the family, which can frequently change. IM physicians must remain alert to red flags that may emerge through these conversations that could disrupt their ability to successfully discharge the patient. Such disruptions have implications for all institutional logics at Pacific Medical Center, so it is critical that discharge management be navigated carefully, safely, and successfully.

On day 3 of her hospital stay, Ms. Farhad's fecal matter continued dripping into her G-tube. Dr. Brandon knew that they had to do something to relieve her impaction. Amina agreed but said that she was worried that treatment could make the patient feel worse: "I think lactulose would be best—giving the best possible chance to clear her out and help her feel better." She discussed possible causes but declared she was unsure why this was happening. Dr. Brandon agreed but said, "I'm not excited to look *too* far with her prognosis." The team then briefly visited Ms. Farhad. Upon leaving the patient's room, Dr. Brandon said, "She looks *much* better today . . . she [was] at death's door when she came in."

Over the course of day 4, the patient continued to improve and had stabilized considerably. It became possible for her to go home. James, another medical student, raised some issues surrounding discharge. He said that Palliative Care wanted a discussion with everyone present—the team and the family—to discuss hospice options.

On day 5 of the patient's stay, the team, who had been on call overnight, gathered in a small office early in the morning to begin morning rounds. Before any discussion of patients could begin, Dr. Brandon said, "*Please* tell me [Ms. Farhad] is going home today!" James at first said no, then laughed: yes, she was going home. A form just needed to be filled out.

Five days later, and to the frustration of the IM team, Ms. Farhad was still in the hospital. The patient's fecal impaction was gradually draining and her overall health had improved considerably after partial parenteral nutrition (PPN) overnight, an enema, and a jejunostomy tube (J-tube).

"Will she be discharged to a SNF [skilled nursing facility]?" asked Dr. Lee, the new attending. Michael told him that a SNF had accepted her, but the family had refused and were just going to take her home. Dr. Lee said, "Okay, tomorrow she goes home." Then, after a brief pause: "That's what *Dr. Brandon* said." The team laughed.

Ms. Farhad remained for an additional five days, resulting in a fifteen-day hospital stay. On day ten, the IM team had been optimistic that the family would be willing to send Ms. Farhad to a skilled nursing facility. Unfortunately, after locating one with an available bed, the family refused, leading to further delays. They ultimately agreed to send her to a rehab center in a nearby affluent neighborhood.

Ms. Farhad's was not a unique discharge case but rather a common occurrence on the IM wards at Pacific Medical Center during my fieldwork. Her extended stay illustrates the complex nature of hospital discharge and the need for physicians to negotiate contradicting pressures of multiple institutional logics. From a health logic perspective, it was crucial to consider Ms. Farhad's health and the risks of a premature discharge or a discharge without adequate follow-up care such as a skilled nursing facility, resulting in an adverse health outcome. Such outcomes can have legal ramifications, making it all the more critical to include the family in decision-making to ensure their satisfaction with care and discharge.

Nonetheless, while striving to achieve these goals a common consequence is delays of care and discharge, jeopardizing the objectives of the hospital's market logic. There are serious financial ramifications for hospitals when patients remain for extended periods without an acute medical need. Furthermore, beyond the single patient, there are patient welfare consequences—other patients who need care cannot be admitted because of a lack of beds. In the case of Ms. Farhad, the medical team had to take into account the patient's age, her family's involvement and their resources, and the severity of her condition. All of this information is significant in whether the IM team privileges the health, market, or legal logic when making discharge determinations.

Sometimes the pressures of conflicting institutional logics are experienced in distinct ways. Other times, the multiple logics align in such a way that a single clinical decision may achieve multiple goals. For IM physicians, the hidden curriculum of doctoring requires figuring out when and how these logics align and how to make decisions that address several needs at once—even if it is at the expense of one logic's goals. For instance, the health and legal logics tend to be aligned but the market logic is neglected. Ms. Farhad's remaining in the hospital for ten additional days had clear financial consequences, but ensuring her safety and that her family was happy had positive health and legal implications. This was a stark contrast to Jordan's quick departure (Chapter 1) and Jessica's (Chapter 3), even though all three patients had very serious health conditions. Variations in discharge decisions show once again how physicians capitalize on the moral polysemy of the health logic—the ambiguity of "patient health and well-being" allows physicians to draw from its different meanings to justify the clinical decisions they make.

Hospital discharge is one of the most complicated aspects of health care delivery at Pacific Medical Center. First and most important, it is extremely unpredictable; even with the best-laid plans, a sudden change in a patient's condition will render them useless. This unpredictability, however, is exactly what drives the IM team to be diligent in establishing a discharge plan and looking out for potential roadblocks.

Roadblocks can come in many forms. Most important, IM trainees quickly recognize that discharge is never a unilateral decision made by the patient's primary care team but rather a careful negotiation across care teams, patients and their families, various specialists, and insurance companies. Successful and timely discharge requires effective (and often repeated) communication with all parties throughout the patient's hospital stay. It also requires knowledge of institutional practices and policies and a familiarity with local health infrastructures because many of the patients at PMC require additional care such as home health services or a skilled nursing facility. Failure to address any one of these issues can lead to adverse patient outcomes, delays of care and discharge, financial losses for the hospital, and risk of legal recourse.

HOSPITAL DISCHARGE MANAGEMENT: CONFLICTING
HEALTH AND MARKET LOGICS

While there are numerous ramifications of poor hospital discharge management, the focus has largely been on how discharge management directly impacts the market logic. Dating back to the late twentieth century, improper hospital discharge management has been touted as a driver of medical waste in the inpatient setting and has therefore been directly targeted in efforts to reduce unnecessary spending. Accordingly, Pacific Medical Center and hospitals across the country have been trying to reduce lengths of stay while ensuring that discharge determinations are safe and effective.

Physicians at PMC are incentivized to quickly discharge patients. However, there are many obstacles to efficient hospital discharge, including unexpected changes in a patient's condition, lack of follow-up care, and patient or family disagreement with a proposed plan. Some of these obstacles are not in the purview of physicians and little can be done to avoid or mitigate them. But others, such as lack of follow-up care, can be prevented. A critical component of the hidden curriculum of doctoring in hospital discharge management is learning how to preemptively identify and address obstacles to avoid discharge delays.

While barriers to hospital discharge may vary from patient to patient, one lesson that all IM physicians quickly learn is that early discharge preparation is vital. The shift toward early discharge planning began in US hospitals in large part because of the 2014 Improving Medicare Post-Acute Care Transformation (IMPACT) Act, established to facilitate effective and economical discharge by preventing complications, adverse health outcomes, immediate readmissions, and improving patient care. Under this legislation, health care professionals would be required to start discharge planning within the first twenty-four hours of hospital admission and fully establish a plan (including follow-up care) prior to the patient's departure that accomplished much more than expedited patient turnover.

A critical complication is that "pushing patients out the door" can deeply compromise their welfare and jeopardize the health logic. Adverse health outcomes and in turn immediate hospital readmissions signal improper management leading to a patient's unstabilized condition or a lack of adequate follow-up care. In order to prevent such missteps, recent changes in insurance reimbursement policies have *disincentivized* quick discharge. Medicare, for instance, penalizes hospitals for what it deems premature discharge evidenced by immediate readmission.[1] These policy changes stem from reports like the one published by the Robert Wood Johnson Foundation in 2013, which announced: "The U.S. health care system suffers from a chronic malady—the revolving door syndrome at its hospitals . . . one in five elderly patients is back in the hospital within 30 days of leaving. . . . Many of these readmissions can and should be prevented."[2] The report placed the onus on health care professionals, claiming that many readmissions were consequences of poor care coordination and insufficient discharge planning.[3] Also in 2013, the federal government exposed the financial stakes of the revolving door syndrome, reporting that "the cost of readmissions for Medicare patients alone [is] $26 billion annually . . . more than $17 billion [of which] pays for return trips that need not happen if patients get the right care."[4] Both reports, combined with the concerted efforts of the Affordable Care Act to minimize unnecessary health care spending via financial incentives,[5] have resulted in conflicting pressures: to expedite hospital discharge and to prevent "avoidable" hospital readmissions

The upshot of the new policies is that PMC and other US hospitals are at financial risk if they keep patients too long *and* if they push patients out too quickly. Thus, it is critical for trainees to learn how to make discharge determinations that ensure patient health and well-being without resulting in penalties for the hospital. Furthermore, not only the health and market logics but the legal logic can be compromised because of mismanagement of hospital discharge. Patient and family perceptions of improper determinations leave both the physician and the hospital open to legal liability. Poor health outcomes associated with immediate hospital readmissions bring into question whether physicians are truly making decisions in the best interest of patients or are overly preoccupied with the financial implications of care.

Although physicians actively negotiate contradictory objectives in patient discharge, they explain their decisions through the lens of the health logic. In this way, they explicitly capitalize on the moral polysemy of patient welfare to justify discharge determinations that are rarely uniform and more often situational. They draw on the hospital's health logic, but they highlight different patient health and well-being factors to rationalize divergent decisions. Some patients are allowed to stay, like Ms. Farhad, and others are forced to leave, like Jessica and Jordan. This lack of uniformity conceals one practice adopted by all IM physicians, however: ensuring patient and family involvement and ultimate satisfaction.

The worst approach to hospital discharge is the primary care team making unilateral decisions without involvement of the patient and family. However, involvement can lead to unexpected challenges if the patient and family are not onboard with the primary care team's plans. To avoid such conflicts, IM physicians carefully craft discharge plans with patient and family input. The IMPACT Act requires that patients' goals be clearly delineated and that patients actively participate in discharge decisions. In 2015, Andy Slavitt, then acting administrator for the Centers for Medicare and Medicaid Services (CMS), commented on a key component of the act: "Individuals will be asked what's most important to them as they choose the next step in their care—whether it is a nursing home or home care. Policies like this put real meaning behind the words consumer-centered health care."[6] CMS deputy administrator and chief medical officer Patrick Conway explained how this new patient-focused policy would work:

> Patients will receive discharge instructions, based on their goals and preferences, that clearly communicate what medications and other follow-up [are] needed after discharge, and pertinent medical information will be communicated to providers who care for the patient after discharge. This leads to better care, smarter spending, and healthier people.[7]

Individual states have begun to apply the IMPACT Act policy changes via statewide programs. For example, California implemented a new discharge policy on January 1, 2016, that states: "The hospital shall provide an opportunity for the patient and his or her designated family caregiver to engage in the discharge planning process, which shall include information and, where appropriate, instruction regarding the post-hospital care needs of the patient."[8] The goal is safer and more efficient discharges as well as fewer disagreements and appeals. Although such policies became mandated largely after my fieldwork ended, PMC was already attuned to them in strengthening and improving hospital discharge and embracing patient and family involvement.

The overall lack of uniformity in hospital discharge determinations reflects their complexities, requiring careful negotiation of multiple moving parts and conflicting objectives. As discussed previously, there are undeniable financial as well as health stakes of both prolonging a hospital stay and prematurely discharging a patient. Legal concerns are also significant, as hasty discharges may lead patients and families to report medical negligence. From a health perspective, patients who remain in a hospital bed prevent others who are truly in need from being admitted. There are implications for the institution's training logic as well: if patients remain in the hospital for prolonged periods without an acute medical need, trainees provide very basic care and so few new learning opportunities arise.

Amidst this complicated context, IM physicians develop specific strategies and tools to achieve safe and effective hospital discharges. The obstacles to appropriate discharge can range from structural to interpersonal. In the following section, I explore the structural obstacles.

GETTING PATIENTS PROPERLY DISCHARGED: ORGANIZATIONAL BARRIERS

Brian, a white man in his twenties, had been admitted to Pacific Medical Center with cardiac issues. After a few days on the Internal Medicine Service, his condition had stabilized to a point that would normally result in departure. However, in Brian's case there was no discharge date in sight because he had no place to go: he was homeless; His girlfriend Samantha was also homeless. The IM team had found a local shelter for him, but he was refusing to go because they would not accept Samantha, who was schizophrenic. He said that he did not want to leave her homeless in her condition. The end result was that Brian remained in the hospital without an acute medical need because his doctors were unable to find a suitable placement option for him and Samantha too.

Brian stayed in the hospital for many days with no sign of leaving until one of the medical students on the team found a shelter that would accept the couple, located approximately one hour away from PMC. During morning rounds, he explained that the shelter was highly selective so he was waiting to hear back from them. The team's spirits were high because the shelter was the first viable option for successfully discharging Brian. It was particularly advantageous because it offered a medical respite program, which provided temporary care and supported recovery for homeless individuals who had recently transitioned out of the hospital.

The medical student was explaining that he would follow up with the shelter, but one of the interns interrupted: "If the patient does go to the shelter, he'll be unable to receive follow-up care at PMC."

"That would be fine since we'll discharge [him] with cardiac medications," the resident said. The intern asked if they could also give the patient oral magnesium so that he could continue treatment at home.

"Is he receiving medications by PO now?" the resident asked.

"[No, but he] could be transitioned to it now," the intern replied.

"That wouldn't be a good idea since he could respond badly to the PO," the resident said. "PO intake of magnesium can lead to diarrhea," the attending explained to the team, which would most likely bring Brian back to the hospital. However, the attending noted that if they did opt to send him home with oral magnesium, they would just "tell him that if he started to get diarrhea, he should stop taking the medication immediately." These instructions would avert a potential hospital readmission due to medication side effects. The intern made note of the plan and the team moved on to the next patient.

Brian's case represents a common discharge dilemma that IM physicians face. Patients end up remaining in the hospital without an acute medical need because of structural factors: primarily institutional practices and policies associated with Pacific Medical Center and the local health infrastructure which prevent discharge. In Brian's case, the rules and restrictions of shelters limited his discharge options.

Brian's case illustrates one of the fundamental organizational barriers to discharge: having nowhere to go, which is especially true for homeless patients because many shelters are overburdened or unable to provide suffi-cient care for the ill. The reality is that hospitals hold onto homeless patients, as one resident noted: "The hospital acts as a shelter, which is such a bad use of resources." Pacific Medical Center is far from alone in this predicament. A 2012 *New York Times* article reported "hundreds of patients . . . languishing for months or even years in New York City hospitals, despite being well enough to be sent home or to nursing centers for less-expensive care."[9]

Even for patients with homes to go to, many of them, like Ms. Farhad, require a higher level of follow-up care than can be provided at home and often need to be transferred to specialized facilities such as a skilled nursing facility (SNF). Physicians must therefore be aware of SNF protocols. For instance, they do not accept patients on weekends, so the IM team must ensure that all transfer paperwork is completed by Friday afternoon at the latest. If not, the patient's discharge is delayed to Monday. Accordingly, time is a critical factor: the earlier physicians and case managers begin to prepare for discharge, the higher the likelihood of an on-time departure.

The ability to prepare is further limited because SNFs and other nursing home facilities typically do not accept a reservation several days prior to dis-charge.[10] Thus, while a case manager can research different facilities and locate an available bed as part of the patient's projected discharge, the bed cannot usually be held. In some cases, when the patient is ready to be discharged the bed that had been available may now be occupied. Unfortunately, insufficient SNFs are a burgeoning concern for hospitals and patients across the country primarily because of a growing aging population. This bed shortage will only be exacerbated without a restructuring of the number and capacity of nursing facilities in the United States.[11] Thus are physicians once again reminded of medicine's market logic as they make outpatient care decisions.

During morning rounds, an intern was presenting a patient who was to be discharged to a SNF. The intern noted that the patient had asked to be discharged with a wheelchair. "[But] if we got him [one], then [he] wouldn't qualify for the SNF that he needs to go to," the resident interrupted. The resident went on to explain that if the patient were to go home and receive home health and physical therapy, he could get a wheelchair, but his insur-ance would not cover one in a SNF. Fortunately, the SNF would provide everything, including the wheelchair, once the patient was admitted. Without such knowledge of the different rules and regulations of insurance companies and external facilities, patients may go without much needed therapies or resources, leading to discharge delays due to denials of coverage, which result in unexpected financial burdens for both patient and hospital.

The inability to secure follow-up care is another common barrier to efficient discharge and, once again, requires physicians to successfully navigate the market logic. Follow-up is crucial because it guarantees that the patient will continue to receive care, protecting overall health and well-being and deterring immediate hospital readmissions. Some patients must have home health personnel accompany them at discharge to set up their homes for outpatient care. This also requires that insurers approve home health and equipment, such as a specialized bed or oxygen, which can delay care and discharge.

One attending recalled a lung disease patient who was ready to be discharged but because it was Saturday he stayed in the hospital until Monday, primarily because he needed to be sent home with oxygen. His insurance was Medi-Cal, which required an ABG (arterial blood gas) test prior to discharge to show the need for oxygen. An ABG test had been performed on Tuesday or Wednesday and by Saturday, the results had expired and the insurer required a new test. The team subsequently scheduled an ABG test on Saturday, but because of the weekend they were unable to secure transportation to send the patient home. To avoid the test expiring *again*, they waited until Monday for the ABG test, which delayed discharge two additional days. This is an example of the careful coordination needed between the primary care team, the patient's insurer, and transportation services, as well as the importance of the IM team scheduling all necessary tests and procedures in anticipation of discharge. Inadequate knowledge of specific insurance coverage rules and restrictions causes repeat testing and discharge delays—two unnecessary costs for the hospital.

PMC physicians also struggle with insurance restrictions and the hospital's market logic when scheduling follow-up care for underinsured and uninsured patients, like Jordan, who cannot receive care at Pacific Medical Center's outpatient offices and so their physicians must find alternatives. Trainees in particular are unfamiliar with the health care landscape and the available care centers for this patient population. Attending physicians and case managers are important resources for trainees in bypassing discharge barriers, teaching them how to secure primary care services for under- and uninsured individuals. One common barrier is the fact that a patient does not have a primary care physician (PCP). However, interns and residents learn that, because they rotate at other medical centers during their residency—specifically those that accept underresourced patients—they can become a patient's PCP. PCP follow-up care is particularly important because outpatient appointments help prevent adverse outcomes, immediate hospital readmissions, and associated financial and legal penalties.

Organizational obstacles to discharge, although challenging, are inevitable given the nature of the US health care system. Most of the IM physicians I interviewed found that with sufficient preparation many obstacles could be quickly addressed. These obstacles stand in stark contrast to interpersonal obstacles, which are a source of extreme frustration for IM physicians. They are the focus of the following section.

REACHING CONSENSUS WITH PATIENTS: INTERPERSONAL BARRIERS TO DISCHARGE

The primary interpersonal barrier to discharge is the inability to reach consensus on a discharge plan with patients and families, as witnessed in Ms. Farhad's case. The goal of consensus aligns with the goals of all four institutional logics. Consensus ensures that patients and families have been included in decision-making and are satisfied with the discharge plan. From a market perspective, it minimizes financial losses associated with improper discharge decision-making, where patients and families are unaware or ill-equipped to manage the discharge plan because of miscommunication. From a legal perspective, consensus can protect against litigation. Patients and families involved in the discharge plan are less likely to allege medical negligence and seek legal recourse for adverse outcomes that emerge post-discharge. Lastly, from a training perspective consensus on discharge is a fundamental lesson for trainees that has direct implications for their education. The ability to turn over patients is critical to acquiring new patients and so learning new clinical skills. While in most cases patients and families adhere to the proposed plan, sometimes this is not the case. *Resistant patients* and their families disagree with the plan, resulting in prolonged hospital stays.

Resistant patients and families can officially contest a discharge by filing a formal appeal with their insurance company. Medicare recipients can have their case reviewed by a quality improvement organization and subsequently be held in the hospital for forty-eight to seventy-two hours while the review takes place. If the evaluation shows in favor of the patient, the patient remains in the hospital; if the evaluation sides with the physician's proposed discharge plan, the patient must leave immediately.

Formal appeals are rare. In the few that came up during my fieldwork at PMC, the patient and family appealed without notifying the IM team. Physicians were often alerted by nurses and case managers during rounds. More commonly, appeals took place informally. Patients and family members might evade discharge-related conversations with physicians and other parties by making themselves unavailable for physician-coordinated meetings, or they might not return physicians' phone calls. Without their participation, consensus could not be reached, impeding successful and efficient discharge. It was often unclear whether busy schedules prohibited forward discussion or family members were ducking phone calls.

Patients and family members also marshal medical knowledge to prove that the patient's stay is necessary, often leading to delays of discharge. They claim that a new symptom has manifested—the patient vomited, had diarrhea, spiked a fever for example—or argue using observational data against a physician's diagnostic or prognostic decision. In some cases, the change in condition is self-evident or documented, but trickier cases come up if symptoms are reported overnight, when physicians and nurses are unable to verify them.

Once vomiting or diarrhea has been reported, physicians and nurses request that future evidence not be flushed down the sink or toilet so it can be assessed. Red flags go up when patients or family members are unable to provide physical evidence because they "accidentally flushed . . . or needed to flush" for others' bathroom use. Nonetheless, even without physical evidence, because these symptoms are medically possible physicians find it difficult to reject them because they could lead to an immediate hospital readmission and even a potential lawsuit.

Family members also present "medical evidence" to convince physicians of an incorrect medical assessment and discharge plan. In one case, family members challenged a medical evaluation and discharge plan. They called the physician to the room because they had observed a change in the patient's condition that they believed justified a longer stay. Upon physical assessment, the attending reported that the patient never tracked with her eyes or squeezed her fingers. The family, however, was convinced that the patient was lucid at times. The nurse tending the patient told the team that, indeed, the patient was lucid, but the nurse had never observed any alertness. The attending explained that the patient was not lucid, that there had been no neurological activity from her for five days, and that the family's belief that the patient was lucid was delaying discharge. The attending told the team that the only solution was for him to bring the family members to the patient's bedside and show him what they believed indicated responsiveness. He also ordered a brain-imaging scan to be completed in order to show the family that she had an altered mental status, as the family's interpretation of a physical change in the patient had led them to defy the physician's assessment.

ENCOURAGING RESISTANT PATIENTS OUT THE DOOR

Physicians see resistant patients as jeopardizing the goals of the hospital's market, health, and training logics. These patients drain the hospital's financial resources, they put themselves at risk for hospital-acquired infections or injuries, they prevent admission of patients in need, and they offer little in the way of medical education. Unsurprisingly, physicians find such patients vexing, especially because the only way to discharge them is to convince them, as well as their families, to adhere to the discharge plan.

Convincing often takes time and a great deal of emotional support. One attending who had completed her residency three months before I interviewed her expressed her exasperation: "You know, the stress of residency can make you irritated and you think, ugh, I have *one* more person to round on. It's *one* more patient to have to deal with." Physicians acknowledge the importance of including patients and families in discharge decision-making, but many convey exasperation when faced with their opposition.

Despite the fact that discharge conversations can be time-consuming, including patients and families improves the discharge process and serves as an opportunity to ensure patient satisfaction and adherence to the objectives of the hospital's health and legal logics. Pacific Medical Center is just one of thousands of hospitals across the country committed to patient satisfaction and acutely cognizant of litigation risks. Partly in response to medical malpractice litigation in the United States, patient satisfaction has become a metric of hospital and physician quality and compensation.[12] This shift has incentivized health care institutions and professionals to meet patients' demands when making care decisions. Studies have found that patient satisfaction relies on factors ranging from services and facilities to involvement in medical decision-making. Pacific Medical Center's commitment to patient satisfaction can be readily seen in its pristine facilities, the numerous amenities offered to patients and families, and the state-of-the-art services it offers.

Furthermore, IM physicians actively engage with patients and families, spending extensive amounts of time with them, particularly those who are distressed and have questions about their care trajectory. Improper or ineffective communication can lead to negative evaluations and, in more extreme cases, litigation. Spending time with patients reduces medical paternalism, promotes effective communication and inclusiveness in decision-making, and builds patient satisfaction and physician trust.[13] Studies have shown that even in incidents of patient harm, rather than the incident itself, patients' and families' perceptions of inadequate communication often lead to legal involvement[14]; patients and families seek legal advice when questions are unanswered and events lack transparency, such as when physicians close ranks.[15]

For such reasons, physicians carefully craft discharge conversations, employing specific strategies to elicit patient compliance. They adopt two basic approaches: marshaling medical knowledge and capitalizing on the involvement of third parties. They use medical knowledge to explain the health risks of unnecessarily remaining in the hospital, showing how the institution's health logic drives discharge determinations. They also present medical data showing that all necessary care was administered and the patient's acute condition was managed; one attending discussed her approach: "I go over the risks of being in the hospital, like infection, clots, a fall, and so forth. I explain what has been done thus far. I go over their concerns." According to another physician,

> The hospital—it's a dangerous place to be in if you don't need to be here. So I try to remind them . . . of the risks of staying in the hospital—like

getting an infection or having some sort of medical error—a nurse could accidentally come into the room and give you a medication by mistake. I just try to tell them that there are many reasons to be in the hospital, but if you don't need to be here—there are risks. . . . I try to come up with a good plan for them going home or wherever they are going to go so that they feel more comfortable with the plan.

All the physicians I interviewed remarked on ways in which the hospital can be a dangerous place, using language that reinforced the health logic as the predominant logic motivating discharge determinations. Physician-led discussions consistently emphasized patient welfare and safety.

In discussions with patients and families, physicians also used the market logic to their advantage. They capitalized on third-party interference by claiming that insurance companies drove discharge plans: if patients were to oppose a discharge date, they would be financially accountable because of insurance restrictions—denials of coverage—which shifted decision-making away from physicians. This rhetoric allowed physicians to adhere to the institution's market logic while also blaming it on the market logic. One physician explained:

And then there are . . . people that really can't tell you why [they want to stay]. They just say, "Well I just want to stay one more day." To those patients you just have to be very clear that you know that when they're ready to go they really need to go. [You tell them] that there's no medical reason to keep them here. We often will tell them too that if their insurance doesn't find an acute medical need for hospitalization that they could end up with the bill because we [the hospital] won't get paid. That often is very motivating . . . for people.

Physicians would also present financial issues as private information that they were disclosing as the patient's ally:

Sometimes they [say], "You guys are just a business, you don't care about me, you're just doing this because of the money." In those cases . . . I'll often say, "I just want you guys to know for *full disclosure*—there's a very good chance that any day after today is not going to be covered [by your insurer]."

By blaming the discharge decision on the financial assessments of third parties, physicians preserved a therapeutic relationship with the patient, emphasizing that their hands were tied by the financial structuring of the system.
This strategy also served the legal logic of the hospital, allowing physicians
to say that financial considerations were not central to physicians' decision-
making but forced on them by third parties.

Discharge discussions become an opportunity to foster patient trust and
counter accusations of profit motive in medicine.[16] Trust is especially important when seeking patient and family compliance and, more broadly, effective
communication. The health communication literature finds that patients' and
families' perceptions of meaningful involvement in medical decision-making
translates into greater trust and satisfaction in the care received despite a
particular health outcome.[17] Therefore, when patients feel included in the
discharge plan, the literature suggests, they will be more comfortable with it.

Patients' and families' disagreements with physicians over discharge elu-
cidate the inherent differentials of power and status in the patient-physician
relationship and leave patients with an uphill battle to be effectively heard,
especially since their inclusion is moderated by physicians. Accordingly,
power and status dynamics will most likely persist, even with patient-centered
care and satisfaction metrics in place. For instance, physicians may adopt
paternalistic attitudes, which patients and families may perceive as their
preferences and perspectives being dismissed as uninformed.[18] Social scientists have found that, when faced with inadequate communication, patients and families depend on actions rather than discussion to voice their
concerns,[19] which might explain some of their behaviors on the IM wards
at PMC, particularly nonverbal cues like avoiding phone calls. According
to researchers who have extensively examined how patients (re)gain power
in medical decision-making—and the patient-physician relationship—such
nonverbal cues are commonly used.[20]

While this research cannot explain resistant patients' true reasons to prolong a hospital stay, some inferences can be drawn. First, fear of health care
professionals and health care settings can be physically manifested. Studies
have indicated that "white coat syndrome" exhibits very real physiological
symptoms, such as elevated blood pressure and heart rate.[21] Unmanaged fear
can therefore result in changes in condition that lead patients to dispute a

discharge decision and even cause physicians to delay discharge to manage symptoms. An 83-year-old woman with diabetes and hypertension who had been admitted to Pacific Medical Center with a UTI and abdominal and back pain, remained in the hospital for fifteen days because the medical team could not determine the cause of her ongoing nausea and vomiting. The team wondered if there were a psychosomatic element involved, given that her vomiting increased after the team discussed her potential discharge. She remained in the hospital because, without further investigation of the clinical cause of her vomiting, she would most likely be immediately readmitted.

Fear may not always manifest as physical symptoms, but it can generate anxiety over leaving the medical personnel and resources available in the hospital after a serious health episode.[22] Attending physicians told me that whenever they were faced with a resistant patient, they first sat down with the patient and family and asked them about any fears and anxieties they had. The attendings tried to assuage these fears and often found that these conversations helped patients and family members feel less apprehensive. While I observed IM teams manage resistant patients and family members on numerous occasions, I much more frequently saw patients and family members simply relinquish discharge decisions to the team.

THE VALUE OF HOLDING PATIENTS

Proper discharge management has largely been understood as timely, appropriate patient departures. However trainees quickly realize the complexities of this process when proper discharge management also includes actively prolonging a patient's hospital stay, regardless of acute care status—thus requiring that they know when *not* to push a patient out the door. In decisions to hold patients seemingly without an acute medical need, IM physicians emphasize the patient's precarious condition and the risk of adverse outcomes from a premature discharge. In such instances, they accept the financial disadvantages of keeping a patient a bit longer than needed from an insurance perspective. Experience and training shape the decision to extend an inpatient stay.

Similar to divergent opinions about consultations, it was common for me to see discharge disagreements between trainees and attending physicians, with trainees tending to advocate discharge and attendings encouraging delay. It is not surprising that trainees are confused and frustrated by the decision to hold patients in certain cases when in other, seemingly similar cases, patients are pushed out. Confusion and frustration are exacerbated by trainees' workloads and their desire to move forward in their training with patients who offer more educational value.

In some disagreements, such as those over clinical care plans, attending physicians may entertain the input of their trainees and alter a treatment course based on their recommendations. However, in discharge disagreements the medical hierarchy usually prevails and the attending's decisions are followed, especially when there may be legal implications. In one such instance at PMC, an intern was discussing a potential discharge for Mr. Kim, a 96-year-old Korean American man who had been admitted to PMC with generalized weakness and severe hyponatremia after falling at home. By day three of his stay, the intern was optimistic that he could be discharged in the afternoon and reviewed the requirements for discharge during morning rounds: twenty-four-hour care at home with his son; follow-up with Urology in the coming weeks; home health every other day; and home physical therapy.

The attending disagreed: "While I'm *always* happy about discharges on my service, I don't think we should go ahead with a definitive discharge [for Mr. Kim]." He explained that Mr. Kim needed to be eating more and that he wanted to see "some stability in [the patient's] sodium levels. If not, he'll come right back so I want to see the sodium increase." The resident and intern agreed to pause their discharge plans and first work on managing Mr. Kim's sodium.

This example reveals that, in order to ensure a safe discharge, the IM team has to be aware of factors that might result in an immediate hospital readmission, which would open the door to financial penalties and a disgruntled, potentially litigious patient and family. In the case of Mr. Kim, the attending physician was concerned that, without continued stabilization of his hyponatremia and increased food intake, he might return to the hospital. While there are no hard and fast rules for discharge decisions, some factors play a more visible role than others.

A patient's condition strongly influences physicians' discharge decision-making. Very sick patients who are stabilized but will inevitably return to the hospital for care due to their condition(s) are granted an extra day, particularly when the patient or the family disagrees with the discharge plan. The majority of physicians I talked to said that they preferred to offer an extra day rather than embroil themselves in a battle over discharge by a given date. One attending explained his reasoning:

> Some patients are so sick [that] you know they are coming back to the hospital . . . two weeks later . . . a month later. And you know that if you give them an extra day and say to the family, "Ok, let's compromise. I'm going to give [your mother] an extra day. We'll see how much oxygen she needs tomorrow. Let's give her some more physical therapy, set her up for outpatient pulmonary rehab." . . . You make some compromises [when] you know that [she'll] back two weeks later and they say, "Oh doctor, good to see you again, thanks for trying to help us but it didn't really work." Whereas if you kick them out one day earlier and say, "No, get out of here—you have no acute medical needs, your insurance company keeps calling me and says we can't take care of you anymore." Then they come back two weeks later and say, "I *told* that doctor she wasn't ready to go and now she's back and she might die because she's even more hypoxemic and it's *all his fault.*"

Physicians justify their decisions not only as in the patient's best interest but also as a way to prevent future patient-physician conflicts and potential legal backlash.

Litigation risk especially encourages physicians to slow hospital discharge and ensure that patients and families are fully onboard with discharge plans. They often calculate legal risk based on conversations they have with patients or families—say a family member initiates a legal discussion of any kind—or if they discover legal or medical professionals are immediate or extended family members. Predictably, an explicit risk of litigation directly translates into an extended hospital stay. As one attending physician explained, "[Patients say], 'I'm not better. . . . If I don't get better . . . and I get readmitted, I'm going to—' not sue necessarily but something along those lines. And if that's the case, then you need to get legal involved." Another attending physician extended a patient's stay for four days after the family involved the legal department. Yet another was hesitant to push discharge because the patient's brother was a medical malpractice lawyer and the patient's sister-in-law was a registered nurse. Collectively, patient condition and legal concerns encourage physicians to capitalize on the moral polysemy of the health logic to justify their decisions.

THE COSTS OF HOSPITAL DISCHARGE

Hospital discharge is an incredibly complex process that requires careful in-teractions with numerous third parties, knowledge of local health infrastruc-tures, effective communication with patients and families, and negotiation of countervailing financial and professional pressures. Discharge entrenches physicians in the broader realities of the current health care system—cost-cutting, bureaucratization, litigation, patient-centered care—burdening them with the difficult task of reconciling the conflicting pressures and divergent outcomes of hospital discharge management: sometimes pushing patients out the door and sometimes keeping patients in.

Physicians become fully aware that their discharge decisions are rarely uniform, as illustrated by patients like Mr. Kim and Ms. Farhad, who remain in the hospital for extended periods, and patients like Jordan and Jessica, who are expected to leave after a few days. These situations are the result of pow-erful yet contradictory institutional logics that force health care practitioners to prioritize different logics at different times. As observed in my fieldwork and discussed throughout this book, at Pacific Medical Center IM physicians regularly make situationally based clinical determinations that seem to lack any standardization (save consultations, where the outcome is almost always calling a specialist) but have a common basis of understanding: all decisions are made with the health logic primarily in mind.

While physicians draw on the health logic to explain and justify dis-charge, nowhere does the market logic feature as prominently and explicitly as it does in discharge management, which if done improperly translates into financial losses for the hospital either through prolonged hospital stays or financial penalties for immediate patient readmissions. With inpatient costs accounting for nearly 30 percent of US health care expenditure, it is hardly surprising that discharge is frequently targeted as a way to stymie unneces-sary spending. A key assumption is that improved discharge management will reduce preventable health care costs, meaning those primarily associated with unnecessary hospital stays.

Indeed, discharge management is critical in inpatient spending, but this book shows that the other aspects of care it discusses—medical notation and consultations—greatly contribute to avoidable inpatient expenditure as well. In the concluding chapter, I explore the unintended costs of the hidden curriculum of doctoring and the dilemmas and conflicts in the clinical setting that have financial consequences not only for the hospital but for the US health care system as a whole.

6 | COSTS

The multiple central yet conflicting institutional logics and a complex intraprofessional work setting create a hidden curriculum of doctoring that IM physicians must navigate at Pacific Medical Center. They are faced with dilemmas and obstacles that directly impact patient care, and as they learn the curriculum they inevitably make compromises that affect the logics' objectives. This book has revealed the various unintended consequences of the hidden curriculum with a focus on its effect on patients' experiences and outcomes. Here I address in more detail another key unintended consequence of the hidden curriculum, which has been briefly discussed throughout the book: the rise in unnecessary inpatient spending.

Unnecessary inpatient expenditure is of particular concern in the US health care system because exponentially rising costs—especially in the inpatient setting—have been a pressing issue since the midtwentieth century and are a trillion-dollar problem today. And yet, despite spending the most on health care in the developed world, the United States performs poorly against basic health metrics, motivating health care professionals and policymakers to continually revisit spending in order to stymie its never-ending growth. The Centers for Medicare and Medicaid Services (CMS) have highlighted four key areas of health care delivery that contribute to the trillion dollars of medical waste: care coordination, overtreatment, administrative complexity, and pricing. Within these broad categories, fragmented care, lack of communication between providers, hospital readmissions, excessive care, defensive medicine, inefficient authorizations and billing, and lack of transparency in pricing are critical contributing factors. CMS's findings demand the question: Why do these problems persist in spite of numerous practice and policy initiatives? What makes health care expenditure in the United States so difficult to contain?

In this book, I have offered some answers to these questions, specifically focusing on inpatient care delivery at an elite academic medical center. Drawing from sociological scholarship, I have demonstrated how the unique organizational structuring of PMC, the multiple conflicting institutional logics, and the intraprofessional dynamics of a shared workplace create an environment ripe with dilemmas and conflicts that deeply challenge care delivery. As physicians learn to negotiate obstacles to care, this process leads to increased expenditure, which has consequences for both patient and hospital. The following sections examine how the institutional environment at Pacific Medical Center encourages seemingly unnecessary inpatient spending.

IS MORE BETTER? RISING COSTS PERPETUATED BY MULTIPLE LOGICS

The health, market, legal, and training logics all create incentives to provide more care, even if it is not necessarily what is best for the patient. This "more is more" culture is a defining feature of US-based medicine that has been largely embraced by both providers and patients. The term "quality health care" has become associated with interspecialty care and advanced medical technologies, which frequently mean both more—and more expensive—interventions. For instance, at Pacific Medical Center there is an institutional expectation that physicians will heavily rely on medical technologies and consultants, meaning more dollars spent. One attending remarked on PMC's aggressive attitude: "If you're a patient at PMC, you'll get a PET scan faster than a chest x-ray"—chest x-rays usually cost hundreds of dollars while PET scans cost thousands. The excessive use of technology is further demonstrated by trainees' care decisions. Whereas interns and residents have become adept at medical workups and interpreting their results, some attending physicians worry that they are more comfortable with scans than physical exams.

As I discussed in Chapter 4, interspecialty care at PMC is associated with high inpatient expenditure. More doctors on a patient's case lead to more procedures and tests. At hospitals like Pacific Medical Center, the scheduling of procedures and tests can be delayed because of the sheer number of patients needing them. Furthermore, coordinating different specialty groups to determine a care plan takes time. One resident said, "There are times when a patient ... ends up staying longer because the consultants are still waiting to talk with our attending and see if from their perspective it's okay for that patient to leave." One IM attending became frustrated when a Gynecology consultant tested a young woman's tumor markers based on a cancer antigen 125 (CA125) blood level measurement of 176. After the workup had been completed, the attending learned that for premenopausal women a CA125 of 200 is considered normal, meaning that this workup was unnecessary and could have been avoided.

More consults and additional workups would be more readily accepted if they resulted in improved health outcomes. Unfortunately, this is not always true: they can lead to worse health outcomes.[1] In a 2014 *Time* article, Dr. Sandeep Jauhar, a cardiologist in New York City, recounted a patient case where interspecialty care led to excessive treatments that did little to improve the patient's health. A 50-year-old, who came to the hospital because of respiratory issues, stayed for a month and received care costing almost a hundred thousand dollars. He was seen by sixteen specialists and underwent twelve procedures yet when discharged showed little improvement in his shortness of breath.[2] While undeniably expensive, if this were a single patient case, it might not have been troublesome, but this is a nationwide pattern, resulting in over $200 billion in inpatient expenditure.[3] Some may argue that medical workups and tests in interspecialty care are profitable for hospitals, but their profits are offset by extended lengths of stay.[4] According to an attending at PMC, "Someone stays for five extra days to get five unnecessary tests and they could have put two more patients in that bed and charged for a DRG [the amount paid per diagnosis] for each one of them."

At Pacific Medical Center, the institutional pressure to call consultants, the desire to maintain collegial relations, and the hierarchical structuring of care delivery in teaching hospitals exacerbate the unintended financial consequences of interspecialty care. IM physicians defer to consultants and their recommendations, even when they think them unnecessary.[5] And it is not just providers and institutional culture that drive "more is better"; patients also play a critical part. As a society, we are uncomfortable with uncertainty, and nowhere is this more evident than in health care. Patients want definitive answers about their condition, therapeutic options, and prognosis, and physicians increasingly yield to their pressure. Physicians are attuned to fulfilling patients' and families' requests because of a commitment to patient satisfaction and patient-centered care delivery.

Patients also have grown more comfortable with a proactive role in medical decision-making, but this does not necessarily change the inherent asymmetry of knowledge between patient and physician,[6] which means that patients' expectations can be misinformed. For example, a 40-year-old woman with a history of recurrent meningitis was experiencing severe abdominal pain and a rash when she was admitted to Pacific Medical Center. Although her symptoms were brought under control, she wished to remain in the hospital despite the IM team's plan to discharge her. During morning rounds, the medical student assigned to the woman's case said about patients like her: "[They] think [if they stay longer] they'll finally get an answer but that's not the case." The attending agreed, noting that no one was talking about her case anymore and it was "considered closed." The resident also agreed: "I think they think that Neuro can answer the question, but I tell them . . . what Neuro says. [They think] there's this special Neuro person who can answer [all their questions]." Patients understandably are afraid and so desire concrete answers about their conditions and prognoses, struggling to accept that a degree of uncertainty will linger even at discharge.[7]

Another contributing factor to "more is better" is physicians' concerns about litigation, which incentivize them to hold onto a therapeutic patient-physician relationship and practice defensive medicine,[8] a consequence of increasing reports of malpractice, negligence, and profit seeking.[9] Unsurprisingly, physicians at Pacific Medical Center are uncomfortable talking about costs with patients and family members, especially when discussing hospital discharge. In the best case, such reticence protects patients and ensures optimal care. The drawback is that when physicians make decisions based on litigation risk, patients are subjected to unnecessary care, which can have physical, emotional, and financial repercussions.[10] Because physicians at PMC strive to meet the conflicting goals of the health, market and legal logics via the hidden curriculum of doctoring, they adopt "more is better" with expensive consequences.

A MISSING CURRICULUM: FINANCIAL TRAINING

The unintended financial effects of the hidden curriculum are exacerbated by IM trainees' unawareness of the financial dimensions of care delivery when they start their residency on the clinical wards. This lack of awareness stems from a pervasive, and persistent, sociocultural belief that medicine and money should remain in distinct spheres.[11] This belief, however, is too simplistic and vastly untrue, as microeconomic sociological scholarship has clearly demonstrated: social, moral, and financial transactions are inextricably intertwined.[12]

Even though financial concerns have always been present in medical care, there is understandable discomfort with seeing health as a commodity to be bought and sold and providers as sellers of health for profit. The unique relationship between patients and doctors, and physicans' intimate access to their patients' physical and emotional states, means that patients are particularly vulnerable. They must have a great deal of trust in their doctors to share private information and comply with "doctor's orders," so any fears of physicians acting in their own interest and not in their patients' are especially problematic.

In the early twentieth century, Talcott Parsons theorized that physicians were institutionally safeguarded from the profit motive and so would never place financial considerations over patient welfare.[13] Later in the twentieth century and in the early twenty-first, we came to recognize that this does not hold true, although the notion that physicians should not be focused on financial considerations remains. Nowhere do we see this more than in the training of medical students and physicians.

The training logic deems most important the guiding of physicians in their education and in their professionalization as physicians. What becomes self-evident in both medical school and residency is that the training logic singularly focuses on the goals and objectives of the health logic: all attention is on medical knowledge and skills, which is wholly appropriate—anything less is unethical. Thus, there is little to no room for formal financial education because of the overwhelming breadth of knowledge that must be covered in medical education. This reflects the cultural approach toward medicine and money. Physicians have been trained not to see costs when providing care, only patient welfare. Yet there are drawbacks to ignoring costs. It quickly becomes obvious that, even if they do not speak of them, physicians are constantly dealing with financial considerations when making decisions on a daily basis with no financial background. In this way, neglecting financial issues in medical training actually hinders care delivery and generates unnecessary inpatient spending.

All of the attendings, residents, and interns I interviewed said that they had had little if any financial training in medical school. They all agreed that this training began through practice in the clinical setting during residency and in early practice as attending physicians.[14] What few lessons were taught stood out in trainees' minds. Here is a second-year resident's recollection of the one and only financial lesson he learned during medical school:

It's not something that has ever been explicitly taught, there's no course in medical school that teaches you this. And maybe that's what we need—a course in medical school just about billing, and just about thinking about expenses. . . . But I remember as a medical student the only time I was really exposed to thinking about how much a treatment cost was when I did a radiology rotation and had to complete one of their assignments. In the radiology office they had a binder of different costs of tests and they told us, 'Okay, think of a diagnosis, look up the radiology that you believe goes along with that diagnosis and then tally up the costs of working it up from a radiographic standpoint.' That was really the only exposure I had to putting dollar signs behind a test."

An intern agreed:

"I don't think anybody learns financial issues [in medical school]—I didn't. Sometimes they give us these tables of what things actually cost the patient, which is nice. It is kind of an eye opener. We get routine labs every morning because you are a hospitalized patient—no other reason. So sometimes they will show us the breakdown of those costs. A liver panel is almost a thousand and routine labs [run] everyday are a couple hundred bucks. They show us that. I think you [also] learn a lot when you have patients that can't get certain tests."

While pricing tables are useful in alerting physicians to the financial repercussions of the decisions they make, encountering patients with financial
restrictions is much more pivotal to their education than formal course work.
The few physicians who had had financial training prior to residency had
to seek it out themselves. A second-year resident explained: "[I was] always
interested in health disparities so I've done research in that area on my own."

There are numerous explanations for the lack of finance courses in formal medical education. First, the extensive biomedical knowledge and skills
that must be mastered within a relatively short time push other aspects of
care to the side. Second, similar to actual clinical practice (not just textbook
learning), medical finance is difficult to teach in a lecture or classroom setting. One attending stated that financial lectures were ineffective and that
encountering financial dilemmas firsthand was the best education: "We did
get some lectures but . . . a lecture is different from . . . actually having to
fill out the billing cards and do all of that yourself." Third, and perhaps
most critical, is the lack of transparency in the financial structuring of care
delivery. Formal financial training is incredibly difficult when it is unclear
what information is "correct" and should be taught. For instance, third-party
payers make billing and costs unclear and inconsistent, with pricing varying
on a patient-to-patient basis because of differences in plans. According to
one attending,

> I never learned about financial issues as a resident. In general, you'll find
> that doctors are very, very poorly educated on finances and the flow of fi-
> nances through a hospital. And to some extent I believe that people don't
> want you to have that information; you can't even find out what it costs
> to take care of someone in a bed on the wards. No one will give you a
> straight answer. [They say], "Well, it depends on the payer, depends on
> the insurance company, depends on the level of nursing, depends on this
> or that."

The fact that standardized pricing and informative billing generally are unavailable to health care professionals is an insurmountable obstacle for those
who wish to become financially informed about the health care system. An
attending I was interviewing said that the lack of financial transparency
made formal training nearly impossible:

I think we need to start educating people on what the different tests cost but nobody knows. I can't do it because I can't quote what a CBC or a Chem 10 lab test costs . . . even though I'm probably more interested in these issues than most people. . . . I would love to be able to quote the numbers and then make a very convincing argument, but I don't think this hospital, or any hospital, has that level of financial sophistication.

According to a second-year resident,

I don't think we really learn any financial stuff in medical school. I'm still very much in the learning phase. I had a patient just now in clinic that I wanted to give a shingles vaccine to. So two weeks ago I had a similar patient that I sent to the pharmacy to pick up the vaccine, and it was going to cost him $250. I sent my patient today for the same thing to see how much it was, and it cost him only $4. How am I supposed to learn this when it doesn't make any sense? I have a patient ask me how much something costs and I have no idea because it completely depends on what their insurance is. . . . It's completely out of my hands.

What are the consequences of physicians' financial ignorance? One attending, who had completed her residency four months prior to her interview, explained that she had never thought about financial issues until a financial crisis emerged for one of her patients:

During my residency training, we had a clinic that was often hard to get into because we were so booked. It could take six to nine months for a patient to be seen for a consult. [Because of this delay] I would push patients to stay in the hospital. One patient was discharged and afterwards received a $78,000 hospital bill under my care. I felt so bad. That was when I began to rethink the idea of maybe not getting labs every day and maybe just rethinking what the "routine" things should and shouldn't be.

A second-year resident in Emergency Medicine learned about the financial side from specific patient cases:

It's unfortunate, but no one trains you for dealing with these types of social economic issues. Med school doesn't prepare you and nor does residency. It's a case-by-case learning experience, and so throughout the years in residency, you see that your seniors become better at dealing with these situations because they've done it before, not because someone has guided them or even told them the rules and regulations on how to deal with these situations.

Clearly, the best education in the financial aspects of care delivery is sustained clinical work. As trainees at PMC spend more time on the wards, they increasingly recognize care decisions and protocols that drive up unnecessary inpatient spending.

Along with clinical experience, superiors—especially attending physicians—play a pivotal role in the financial education of trainees. An attending emphasized this role:

> I think that in terms of other financial issues that come up there are certainly times when some choices are made by the housestaff in terms of . . . certain types of medications that they are more familiar with but may not be the most cost-effective choice . . . and that's something where the attending physician should certainly suggest to the housestaff that there are other options."

_____

Growing experience on the clinical wards helps trainees recognize how routine care, such as tests, procedures, and consultations, lead to unnecessary inpatient spending. For instance, they realize that tests and procedures are frequently delayed at PMC because of an overload of patients. Through this routine backlogging, they learn which tests should be scheduled first when several have been ordered. For example, when a patient needs both PET and MRI scans, the PET scan is always scheduled first since the waiting list is long and constantly disrupted with emergent cases that are given priority. In addition, many tests and procedures require technicians, who are not available on nights and weekends (except in emergent situations), meaning that patients must stay overnight or through the weekend.

A crucial realization for trainees is that testing begets more testing and a single abnormal reading requires more evaluation. More testing is to be embraced if it leads to valuable new information that changes the patient's care trajectory, but this is incredibly rare. Instead, trainees find themselves chasing a single abnormal test result with more tests and more medical workups, with no change in the patient's condition or care plan.

My interviewees told me that complete medical workups were standard at PMC even though unnecessary and financially costly for the hospital. One resident challenged the hospital's reliance on lab work: "I don't do daily [morning] labs for patients being discharged the same day. These labs find reasons for [a patient] to stay." Many residents adopted this approach.[15] However while this strategy is useful, in some cases labs simply cannot be skipped, which brings to mind the unpredictable nature of biomedicine and the human condition.

Consultations also result in increased inpatient costs—many perceived as avoidable. IM physicians struggle with bringing additional specialists onboard, which is usually accompanied by new tests, procedures, and time-consuming workups. An attending explained:

> [When we call] consultants, especially if we get them involved later in the hospitalization, they don't know the patient from the beginning, they don't have a good feel about what's going on, so they order a whole bunch of tests and procedures, and that, inevitably, delays everything. And things really slow down over the weekend, so if you get a consultant involved on Friday and they recommend these different things that can't be done over the weekend, then right there is at least an additional two-day stay.

In these instances, there is nothing the IM team can do but wait. Delays, however, do encourage careful deliberation before orders are placed.

Rather than officially call a specialist, IM physicians occasionally conduct a "curbside consult," which a trainee who had just begun his second year of residency described:

> A curbside consultation I liken it to a family member or friend asking me offhand, "I have a coworker who has X, Y and Z. What do you think it is?" That's the idea of a curbside. The consultant doesn't physically see the patient, doesn't physically do a chart review of the patient's medical history, may not have the full facts and full picture of the patient. It's just . . . the patient has X, Y, and Z symptoms. They're on X, Y, and Z medications. What do you think is going on? What do you think we should do? If I'm not sure if I'm making the right clinical decisions, I ask the consultant if my decision is okay. When you curbside a consultant, it's yes or no.

"Yes, I would do this. No, I would do something else. This is what I would do." So it's not a full consult.

Sometimes the IM team will call a consultant immediately to evaluate and follow the patient as early as possible. Time can be a tricky thing, however, and there are situations when the team calls a consultant *too* quickly. Inefficient and unnecessary consultations also arise when IM physicians call a consultant with insufficient information about the patient's condition. The upshot, again, is unnecessary tests and procedures and thus delays in gaining a better understanding of the patient's acute needs.

While there is an expectation that trainees will learn to provide financially savvy care through clinical practice, they receive mixed messages on its importance. Trainees I interviewed said they were rarely evaluated on their ability to provide cost-effective care (even though attendings felt housestaff *should* be evaluated on this). Thus, although many attendings commented that trainees were largely unable to provide financially smart care, they were lenient in their few financial assessments, showing that assessments, positive or negative, were of little consequence to the professional trajectory of housestaff. According to the socialization literature, however, evaluations are critical in teaching trainees the expectations, values, and behaviors held in highest regard by the medical profession.[16] In this way, they are socialized to position financial concerns far below other professional responsibilities.

Disregard for finances may seem warranted, and even ideal, if the trade-off is patient well-being. However, physicians who fail to recognize the financial costs of the decisions they make may leave patients choosing to forgo care or render them destitute when the bills come due. The physical and emotional strain of both health and financial concerns accelerates the likelihood of poor health outcomes.

While many support the premise that medicine and money should remain distinct in the name of patient welfare, I argue that this is a fundamentally wrong approach to care delivery that actually jeopardizes the health and well-being of patients and leads to unnecessary medical waste for the health care system. The reality is that the IM physicians at Pacific Medical Center are reminded daily of the interconnectedness of the health and market logics in clinical care. They also see how the legal and training logics directly impact the care decisions they make. Accordingly, rather than trying to fight the realities of the current system and shielding trainees from harsh truths, physicians must embrace the hospital's logics, which they are already forced to do on the clinical wards, and integrate them as early as possible in their training to minimize critical errors and obstacles due to a lack of knowledge or the failure to deal with multiple, conflicting logics.

CONTRIBUTIONS TO THE STUDY OF PROFESSIONS AND ORGANIZATIONS

My focus on the emergence of a hidden curriculum of doctoring on the inpatient wards places this book in the extensive literature that examines the socialization and professionalization of physicians.[17] This literature elucidates the professional and personal challenges all trainees encounter—the rites of passage—as they progress through training.[18] Of particular interest to medical sociologists is the unmasking of the hidden curriculum, which informally socializes and professionalizes medical trainees,[19] shaping their values,[20] actions,[21] and perceptions of both medicine and the medical profession.[22]

Numerous scholars have studied how the socialization and professionalization of physicians during their formal medical training[23] reinforces their professionalism.[24] For instance, in the seminal work *Boys in White*, Becker et al. (1976) explained how medical students manage the professional expectations of "being a doctor," which include mastering an almost insurmountable breadth of medical knowledge and managing anxieties and other emotions in order to impress their superiors. Renee Fox (1957) and Donald Light (1979) documented how physicians-in-training learn to cope with the uncertainties and limitations of biomedicine.[25] In his ethnography of surgical residency, Charles Bosk showed how error management socializes residents to learn the moral values of the medical profession.[26] Firsthand experiences with autopsies[27] and terminal patients[28] are two examples that demonstrate how novice physicians become emotionally socialized in order to provide objective and empathetic care.

The studies just mentioned lay bare the transformation physicians-in-training undergo. Both formal and informal lessons imbue students with new perspectives on what it means to be a doctor—which are often in stark contrast to the perspectives they held on their first day of medical school.[29] Absent in the literature, however, is how physicians learn to practice medicine within a highly specialized, commodified, and bureaucratized health care setting.[30]

This book has contributed to the medical sociological scholarship by revealing the hidden curriculum of doctoring in the inpatient setting which teaches trainees how to provide care in the current health care environment. Drawing on microeconomic sociology's extensive work on organizations, it has shown that Pacific Medical Center, like other elite academic medical centers, is a hybrid organization defined by multiple conflicting yet highly central institutional logics. At PMC, the four institutional logics I have dealt with here—health, market, legal, and training—create a microcosm of the larger health care system. Once on the clinical wards, IM physicians immediately encounter macrolevel policies and pressures that characterize health care delivery in the United States today, including concerted efforts to address rising costs, promote patient centeredness, and minimize litigation risk.

The hidden curriculum of doctoring reveals how complex pressures are often contradictory, forcing IM physicians to recognize that there are rarely straightforward solutions to the challenges that arise. Instead, these challenges require careful consideration and negotiation of countervailing pressures without which improper management of care delivery will lead to compromised care and unnecessary health care spending.

Drawing on the concept of moral polysemy, this book has furthered understanding of how highly central and contradictory institutional logics and complex intraprofessional dynamics directly shape the ways in which individuals make sense of their work on the ground. I have shown that the moral polysemy of the health logic allows IM physicians to make clinical decisions that address multiple institutional needs. Resonating with the work of Altomonte (2020), my work has shown how physicians justify vastly different clinical decisions—particularly around hospital discharge.

I have also revealed, however, that not all decisions are situationally produced, specifically those in hospital consultations. While physicians draw from the moral polysemy of the health logic to justify interspecialty care, the outcome remains uniform: consultants are routinely called and their recommendations are heeded. Here we see how structural factors directly constrain the agency of individual actors: Pacific Medical Center's institutional culture and professional work dynamics force IM physicians to share patients with specialists even when interspecialty care is unnecessary. By capitalizing on the multiple meanings of the health logic, physicians meet the ethical and professional expectations of their profession while working within the constraints of a highly commodified, specialized, and bureaucratized system.

Along with new curricula pivotal to trainees' socialization and professionalization, I have expanded the conceptualization of the trainee, which usually refers to a medical student, intern, or resident. I have shown how critical learning continues beyond residency and during the early years of practice as an attending physician. The training process—and subsequent socialization and professionalization—begins in medical school and residency and continues into early practice as attendings, with individuals facing crucial dilemmas and lessons at different professional stages.[31]

DIFFERENT CONTEXTS, DIFFERENT PRESSURES

From both the literature and anecdotes, we know that health care settings differ vastly, Health care institutions are directly shaped by their patient population, financial structuring and funding, community setting, size, and so forth. Reich's (2014) examination of the commodification of care at three hospitals in the western United States concluded that a hospital's historical roots and patient population directly influence how universal market pressures are experienced by health care providers. According to Reich, the commodification of care, with its bureaucratization and its cost-cutting initiatives, takes on divergent meanings and in turn diverse practices and policies. These directly shape health care professionals' experiences, including their inter- and intraprofessional interactions, their relationships with patients, and even their compensation and benefits. Each institutional context impacts the pressures, dilemmas, and challenges that physicians must learn to navigate.

As one would expect, then, health care training is heterogenous, with trainees having very different experiences based on where their training takes place. For instance, community hospitals, where more than 75 percent of medical residency programs are located,[32] frequently have fewer resources than university hospitals.[33] Furthermore, their residents work independently far more often.[34] Indeed, in my research residents who primarily trained at a county hospital and rotated occasionally at PMC told me that the problems they typically faced at their home hospital were different from those at PMC.

They found themselves frequently isolated, making decisions with few opportunities to obtain advice or help from superiors. There were fewer learning opportunities with an entire team, unlike at PMC, where team learning was integral to the residency program; instead, they were forced to wear different hats—physician, social worker, discharge planner—with each patient they saw. These differences support Jenkins's (2018) work on the heterogenous and stratified experience of residency training in the United States, where even in the same training program at the same institution residents' experiences become stratified and lead to different learning trajectories.

The heterogeneity of medical training in the United States further reminds us that at completion of training physicians find themselves in extremely different contexts of practice that directly define the daily pressures, dilemmas, and challenges they face in their day-to-day provision of care. Thus, it is important to note that this book has highlighted a *specific* subset of challenges faced by residents at an elite university hospital, and in actuality, there is a broader multiplicity of challenges that they may face based on the type of institution they practice in. Where a physician ultimately practices medicine is shaped by factors both personal and professional.

Specialization is a professional factor that has a deep impact on practice context. For instance, primary care practitioners are more likely to practice in underserved rural areas with fewer resources. They are also more likely to see Medicaid and other underresourced patients.[35] The patients doctors see directly translate into the dilemmas they encounter—particularly those shaped by market and legal considerations.

From the late twentieth century to the present, much of the medical sociological literature has focused on the role of patients in health care encounters, zeroing in on their identities, practices, and agency, and labeling them as consumerist, empowered, and engaged.[36] Regardless of label, there is an assumption that patients are increasingly proactive in their own health and health care, with greater responsibility to monitor their health, seek out medical care, be savvy health consumers, and so forth. For instance, Gengler (2014) explored how parents navigate care for children diagnosed with life-threatening conditions at an elite medical institution. Drawing on the concept of cultural health capital, she reported that parents tended to enter one of two distinct trajectories of care engagement: captaining and entrusting. Care captaining included "negotiating with health care providers, conducting sophisticated research on available doctors, hospitals, and treatments, and successfully intervening to influence the care their children received."[37] These parents had high cultural health capital and were unafraid "to hold key actors accountable . . . when they deemed [it] necessary."[38] In contrast, care-entrusting parents left the medical decision making to physicians, resulting in immensely different care and illness experiences within the same medical institution. Like training experiences and health care institutions, there are great variations across patient populations.[39]

Patients' abilities to adopt proactive, consumerist, engaged, or digitized practices in health care delivery depends on the resources available to them.[40] In particular, elderly, underinsured, and minority patients are disproportionately disadvantaged by the heavy reliance on information technologies in health care exchanges. In my time at Pacific Medical Center, I saw a fair number of engaged patients and families who required IM physicians to share clinical decision-making with them. However, not all institutions will have many such patients. Some have primarily patients who seek, or simply have no other option than to accept, paternalistic or care-entrusting health care exchanges. In such instances, physicians may not face the same challenges, such as in discharge management, encountered regularly at PMC. There may also be fewer legal concerns when patients accept paternalistic care and are without the resources to pursue remedies in instances of conflict with the health care team or institution.

Nevertheless, with underserved populations there may be other critical dilemmas, such as patients' and families' concerns regarding the financial implications of care decisions. At PMC financial issues typically arose with discharge management, not usually inpatient care decisions. In other hospital settings, patients and families may regularly reject treatment recommendations and plans because of their cost. To an even greater extent than at PMC, physicians in underresourced patient settings must learn how to effectively provide care to patients with limited resources.

In a similar vein, during my fieldwork at PMC I often observed IM physicians negotiating extended hospital stays; in other inpatient settings, physicians may need to work hard to convince patients to remain in the hospital to receive necessary treatment. Furthermore, some may encounter the "less is more" approach to care more frequently than the "more is more" approach preferred at Pacific Medical Center, again shifting the pressures and dilemmas that physicians face day to day. These variations in health care contexts and exchanges with different patient populations reveal the numerous hidden curricula physicians deal with when they begin to practice medicine on their own.

THE US HEALTH CARE SYSTEM: IS CHANGE POSSIBLE?

The fragmentation and extensive variation in clinical settings in the US health care system, unsurprisingly, make it difficult for policies to translate into effective change. One concern dating back to the twentieth century has been the nation's poor health outcomes compared with its OECD counterparts, in spite of exorbitant spending. The growth of new professional groups, like hospitalists in the 1990s, changes in health insurance reimbursement plans, such as DRGs in the 1970s, new Medicare policies in the early 2000s, and sweeping legislative changes, specifically the 2010 Patient Protection and Affordable Care Act—all of these "solutions" have been implemented to fix a broken system, with special attention to its high costs.[41] Across these strategies, a commonality is the focus on hospital care, especially discharge.

Discharge and readmission have been significant health care issues since the 1990s and remain the topic of policy and clinical conversations in large part because of research findings such as from the 2008 *Dartmouth Atlas* report, which revealed the high cost of variations in treatments and lengths of stay for the same condition across US hospitals.[42] What was especially concerning was that the hospitals that utilize the most resources, keep patients the longest, and spend the most money do not necessarily deliver the best care. Similarly, research conducted by the Robert Wood Johnson Foundation and the Centers for Medicare and Medicaid Services point to improper hospital discharge planning as a major financial drain on the system.[43] The result has been a focus on policies and programs to rein in unnecessary inpatient spending.

Unfortunately, even with decades of policy changes inpatient spending continues to rise, revealing that concerted efforts to target hospital care to date have fallen short of their goals.[44] This book has shed light on the tendency toward failure because of critical organizational and professional factors that affect the decisions clinicians make. These are the specialization of medicine, the commodification and bureaucratization of care, the rise in patient-centered care, and the risk of litigation.

RECOMMENDATIONS FOR PRACTICE

Policy efforts in any field, but especially in health care, are exceedingly difficult because of the system's complex structuring and its many moving parts.
For instance, from a sociological perspective there is a critical flaw in current
cost-cutting initiatives, particularly those dealing with hospital discharge
and readmission: they have been reduced to a numbers game. In line with
the broader movement toward standardization in medical care in the United
States,[45] evaluation and penalization of hospitals is contingent on numerical
data on average lengths of stay and readmissions for individual hospitals.
Standardized care privileges scientific evidence, usually in the form of statistical data, to shape how care is administered. However, by focusing on metrics,
evaluation ignores the broader social context in which a series of decisions
determines why a patient remains in, or leaves, a hospital.[46]

This book has highlighted important local and broader structural factors that directly affect care delivery and the implementation of frequently
adopted practice and policy recommendations, often created from the top
down and conceived without a full understanding of the complexities of the
clinical setting. I have revealed how these complexities directly influence
clinical decision-making, making it difficult to generate policy changes that
will unambiguously improve the current system.

Nonetheless, the system's persistent shortcomings require reform, for as
Kaufman (2015) so aptly stated in *Ordinary Medicine*, our current approach,
one that is "dominated by market priorities . . . [and shaped by] the primacy
of individual rights (but only for those who have gained access to the system),"
can have dire consequences for our society.[47] She asked whether "[we will]
continue to allow the enterprise to be organized and driven by profit and
market share . . . [or is] there a way to turn the cultural rhetoric away from
individual rights and toward the public good?"[48] While perhaps not able to
fully address these questions, this book has offered insights that point to
practice and policy reform opportunities.

First, and most important, it is clear that physicians are the gatekeepers to
both quality care and inpatient costs. Yet, as Kaufman (2015) explains, doctors
are also "downstream from the transformations that frame treatment decision making in the first place, and they must function within the pressures,
values, and politics that undergird the health care enterprise." Resonating
with Kaufman's examination of the driving factors and consequences of the

"more is better" approach, this book has revealed how physicians are on the one hand gatekeepers, and on the other hand are constrained to make clinical decisions that are not always in line with their preferred judgment. With this in mind, the book has ultimately revealed, once again, how critical physicians are on the ground in clinical decision-making and in the consequences of the decisions made. Therefore, quality improvement and cost reduction policies should continue to target doctors and their practice.

Still, it is equally important to recognize that physicians are indeed downstream of the many factors that directly affect their decisions. In particular, they are immersed in highly specialized and highly bureaucratized health care settings that are affected by broader sociocultural, financial, and political processes. Accordingly, it is essential to address the organizational factors that have direct implications for professional experiences and consequently for health care quality and costs. Given the broad variation in health care settings, however, there will never be a policy or practice recommendation that can be uniformly applied. Nonetheless, this book has pointed to changes that might lift some of the current system's burdens. With this in mind, I offer three policy recommendations for both practitioners and organizations.

Introduce the Market Logic in Medical Training

Medical schools and the majority of residency programs remain focused on mastering clinical knowledge and skills, which is understandable given the sheer scope of biomedical knowledge.[49] However, disregarding financial restrictions and constraints on clinical decision-making is impractical. Learning to make decisions that account for financial realities must be incorporated into daily training in a more formal way.

Attending physicians and case managers are valuable resources, but more must be done to improve trainees' understanding of these realities—informal lessons and trial and error cannot be the primary modes of financial education or patients will suffer. If the financial aspects of care delivery can be incorporated into the formal medical curriculum through coursework, clinical rotations, and enforced evaluations, trainees will develop a stronger basis for navigating them as residents.

One evaluation approach is to include a follow-up care plan component to simulated patient case exams.[50] Along with a patient's diagnosis and immediate treatment plan, a component of the evaluation would be a follow-up care plan based on the patient's financial status. In addition, evaluation of trainees' knowledge of the financial aspects of care delivery must be more stringent in their residency. Over the course of my fieldwork, PMC's Internal Medicine Service implemented informational sessions on the social dimensions of care—consultations, financial costs, and so forth. However, there was little information on and assessment of improper management of these social and financial dimensions in care, which is especially concerning for IM physicians, as this information is critical to patient welfare and hospital functioning.

The social and financial dimensions of care delivery should be incorporated into the formal curriculum during medical school and residency with explicit evaluations. Current training, with minimal evaluations, sends the opposite message: the social and financial dimensions of care delivery are of little consequence to trainees' growth as health care professionals.

Strengthen Hospital and Outpatient Facility Networks

Transitions of care out of the hospital are the largest and most costly obstacles to discharge. They can be overcome by strengthening regional health infrastructures,[51] such as by improving ties between hospitals and local clinics and placement centers to allow physicians to quickly learn affordable care options for underresourced patients whose discharge is delayed because physicians are unable to place them. Some US hospitals are reducing lengths of stay and readmission rates by establishing observation units that allow hospitals to house patients without officially admitting them—as outpatients they are not included in data on average lengths of stay and readmissions. Unfortunately, while there is some indication that observation units may actually save money,[52] only a third of US hospitals have them, making this a difficult policy change to implement universally.

Some hospitals have begun to rely on postdischarge clinics located on-campus or nearby where, according to Beresford (2011), patients "can be seen once or a few times . . . to make sure that health education started in the hospital is understood and followed, and that prescriptions ordered in the hospital are being taken on schedule."[53] Hospitals in Boston, Seattle, and Tallahassee, have postdischarge clinics and have reported decreased rates of readmission.[54] Generally, there is strong evidence that secure follow-up care options improve patients' health and dramatically decrease readmission costs.

Partnerships like those just described, which will ideally restructure financial resources within the local health infrastructure, may also help with the current lack of beds in US nursing homes. In 2019 Healy reported that rural nursing homes across the nation have been closing because of insufficient funds.[55] These closures are becoming increasingly common in areas with already inadequate health resources, putting patients at higher risk for greater morbidity and mortality. It is critical that nursing homes and other transitions-of-care facilities be financially supported because without them patients have no place to go after discharge and in many cases are sheltered in hospitals. What are the consequences of this? A 2012 *New York Times* article reported that "care for a patient languishing in a hospital can cost more than $100,000 a year, while care in a nursing home can cost $20,000 or less." In New York, three hundred unplaced patients are known to have stayed in a hospital for up to five years,[56] costing $2 million each year. Such realities point to larger ethical questions about the ability of a health care system to meet the needs of a nation if it continues to generate massive waste and exponentially increasing expenditures.

Start National Campaigns to Minimize Unnecessary Care

While care delivery is shaped by an organization's culture, many practices and policies—from testing to discharge planning—are shaped by research that determines best practices, cultural approaches to medicine ("more is better"), and a health care landscape that cultivates defensive medicine and fragmented care. Largely universal practices and policies become embedded in institutions across the country simply because "this is how things are done." Accordingly, shifting national practices and approaches to care will undoubtedly have an impact at the organizational level.

For instance, in recent years there has been increased scrutiny of physicians' "routine" ordering of tests. In direct response, the resident-initiated *Think Twice, Stick Once* campaign was begun at the University of California, San Francisco Medical Center in the summer of 2014.[57] In a 2018 *Los Angeles Times* article, an ER physician lamented the current culture in medicine, stating that there are "few barriers to ordering tests, which are generally perceived as efficient, remunerative and a safeguard when it comes to avoiding or winning lawsuits."[58] Doctors "may see testing as a way to bypass the hard work of explaining health care decisions" but it is not just physicians driving the testing culture, however; patients play a key role as well, "encouraged by drug and health care marketing [to have] unreasonable expectations about what medicine can offer."[59] Thus, a "just to be safe" attitude develops, "conveying a reassuring sense of caring and patient advocacy on the part of the doctor while also implying, de facto, that the benefits of testing outweigh the dangers."[60] IM physicians at PMC struggle with a slew of supposedly routine tests and procedures that are often automatically performed in collaboration with consultants.

Reevaluating protocols and introducing policies to minimize excessive care are examples of change that will benefit patients, physicians, the hospital, and the larger health care system. As with quality improvement, a focus specifically on medical errors and patient safety protocols should be instituted, driven by task forces to examine and revise best-care protocols across medical conditions and medical specialties with emphasis on unnecessary care. Concerted effort will result in many new programs like *Think Twice, Stick Once* that will not only improve the quality of care but also minimize avoidable medical waste. Furthermore, pilot programs at academic medical centers like PMC, which as research institutions are accustomed to clinical and practice innovations, will allow for testing of efficacy and determining the feasibility of implementing such programming on a national scale.

While my proposals cannot fix all shortcomings of our health care system, perhaps they can change the direction in which we find ourselves perpetually heading when it comes to health care in the United States. Looking to more upstream solutions, such as medical education and training, national programs, and reconfigured local health care networks, may encourage medical professionals to engage in care on the ground that at the very least lessens rather than exacerbates the problems of the current system.

ARE THESE CONTEXTS AND DILEMMAS US-SPECIFIC?

It is universally known that the US health care system, with one of the highest health care expenditures in the world, is unique. A common critique centers on its complicated financial structuring and high fragmentation. The federal government, managed care companies, the pharmaceutical industry, and other third parties—all shape how care is provided and how much it costs,[61] undoubtedly complicating the dilemmas that IM physicians confront on the wards at Pacific Medical Center. Unlike the United States, other developed nations have organized their health care systems as single-payer with the government as the primary regulatory body. This model understandably alters the nature of care delivery and the dilemmas that providers may encounter. Nonetheless, I would argue that the dilemmas IM physicians face at PMC are not so far afield from the concerns health care practitioners must grapple with in other countries.

Similar to the experiences of IM physicians at PMC, ensuring high-quality care like proper care coordination and hospital discharge while minimizing expenditures is a persistent trade-off for practitioners around the world. In England, the National Health Service oversees the health care system and controls the budget.[62] But even with fewer entities in the system, care coordination remains a critical issue. The 2012 UK Health and Social Care Act pushed for greater integration of hospital- and community-based health services.[63] Furthermore, because the NHS has a global budget that cannot be exceeded within a three-year cycle, providers are expected to make cost-benefit analyses in care decisions, which has unfortunately led to compromised care.[64] In Canada, provinces and territories are largely responsible for organizing and delivering health services and supervising providers.[65] Costs are largely controlled through single-payer purchasing and global budgets for hospitals and regional health authorities, but concerns persist. Since 2015, the campaign Choosing Wisely Canada has provided recommendations for reducing unnecessary care.[66]

In Japan, the government regulates nearly all aspects of its universal public health insurance system (PHIS). In recent years, care coordination has been prioritized, with financial incentives for hospitals and clinics to provide effective postdischarge care that adheres to follow-up protocols.[67] In addition, the government implemented the Cost-Containment Plan for Health Care to promote healthy behavior and reduce spending. In particular, health care professionals have been directed to carefully manage lengths of stay and use generic substitutions when prescribing medications.[68] Similarly, in Singapore, where the government maintains the nation's public health care system,[69] hospitals are given annual budgets so they are aware in advance of reimbursements: each year they must break even.[70] Accordingly, practitioners must carefully evaluate their care decisions to ensure that they do not exceed their financial allotment.

In sum, while health care systems are structured very differently around the globe, dilemmas of cost containment and quality care are universal;

providers are expected to make difficult decisions that weigh cost versus care and outcomes. While the United States is indeed unique, the tensions between care and costs emerge in health care systems throughout the world.

CONCLUSION

The hidden curriculum of doctoring is a crucial, and inevitable, aspect of learning that all physicians encounter through clinical practice. Some are fortunate to begin grasping the realities of health care delivery toward the end of their medical school training. Others are navigating and negotiating these realities, which stem from a highly specialized, commodified, and bu-reaucratized system, as novice attendings. Nonetheless, all physicians must grasp the realities of practicing medicine in the United States in the twenty-first century. It is crucial that physicians be supported because the learning curve they must ascend has implications for quality of care and patient welfare as inpatient spending accelerates. To "do no harm" does not mean to ignore all that is "external" to patient health and well-being. "Do no harm" requires that physicians learn to balance the often contradictory values in a health care system that is highly commodified, bureaucratized, specialized, and patient-centered.

Appendix: Methods

The ethnographic[1] fieldwork for this book took place at Pacific Medical Center, a highly specialized, teaching hospital in the western United States. I entered the field with some good luck in September of 2010. I gained access to the Internal Medicine Service at PMC by joining a research team planning to examine the dynamics of end-of-life care. Prior to this, I had been searching for over two years for a field site. At the time, my interests were broadly related to medical decision-making, uncertainty, and the commodification of care. I had met with oncologists to discuss studying tumor boards and had conducted some preliminary observations of physician-patient interactions at an orthopedic hospital, but neither research opportunity panned out. My struggles reflect the common methodological concern of gaining physical access to a field site.[2]

Further complicating this process were unique challenges to "studying up" as well.[3] When attempting to study elites, physical access is particularly difficult because elites tend to establish barriers that "set their members apart from the rest of society."[4] There are often gatekeepers "who keep an eye on the comings and goings of strangers,"[5] as they are accustomed to privacy while at work.[6] Numerous ethnographers have described the arduous process of gaining access, highlighting the challenges they faced and the strategies they used to bypass these barriers.[7]

Upon joining the end-of-life research team, I was fortunate to be included in negotiations to gain access to the Internal Medicine Service at PMC. I attended numerous meetings with various physicians to discuss the merits of my project and ethnographic approach. We presented the proposed research plan and fielded any and all questions or concerns. We were also very fortunate that Dr. Brandon, director of hospitalists, was interested in ethnographic research and the idea of approaching clinical care from a sociological perspective.[8] While negotiations took about three months (as multiple meetings were required with highly placed administrators for approval), Dr. Brandon's support of my proposed research facilitated success.[9]

Once on the wards, I began preliminary data collection with another member of the research team. Internal Medicine was an ideal setting because it was a general service: it admitted a broad range of patients and many of them were elderly. Dr. Brandon, our primary contact person, introduced us to the various IM teams and attending physicians (in person or via email). Like many researchers however, once in the field I shifted direction. Specifically, I branched out from the team to explore a new inquiry: therapeutic decision-making. I was particularly interested in how physicians made clinical decisions when there was no clear "best protocol" for care or for the consequences of these decisions. Furthermore, I was especially interested in how and when physicians determined the best course of action when there were conflicting options. Recall, for example, Ms. Johnson, who needed a surgical procedure but in order to have it was taken off of her blood thinner, which unfortunately led to a stroke. Such cases led me to a new question: How do doctors make medical decisions when faced with incredibly murky clinical situations?

As I spent more time on the wards, I realized that such decisions were not necessarily the most significant for physicians in their daily work. Rather, much of their time was spent grappling with intraprofessional disputes, third-party interference, and financial and bureaucratic constraints. Thus, I once again shifted my research topic. Yet there was a common thread across my two points of inquiry: the everyday decisions IM physicians had to make were incredibly difficult and the solutions were rarely straightforward. They constantly needed to weigh benefits and drawbacks, when to make concessions and when not to. What quickly emerged through my data was that this knowledge was crucial to the socialization and professionalization of physicians, exposing trainees and novice attendings to the realities of care delivery in the current health care landscape.

IN THE FIELD

I was in the field for a total of twenty-six months, collecting ethnographic and interview data on the IM wards at Pacific Medical Center from September 2010 to August 2013 and from mid-July to mid-August of 2015.[10] My ethnographic observations took place primarily during morning rounds and occasionally during afternoon interdisciplinary rounds. There were six IM teams that oversaw all patients at Pacific Medical Center, comprising an attending physician, a resident, two interns, and one or two medical students. Each team had an equal chance of being observed at first, but as I got to know some attendings better, I tried to observe their teams regularly.

Dr. Brandon provided me with the wards schedule and contact information for the attendings. Based on the schedule, I directly emailed the attendings and asked to observe. If I received no response, I waited outside the rounding room—an office space of sorts for trainees and where teams typically met before rounds—and approached the first attending to arrive. I explained the project and my methodology of participant observation. If the attending agreed to participate, I presented the project to the rest of the team. If they consented to the study, I would then proceed to shadow the team from Monday thru Friday. In some instances, I would only conduct observations two to three days of the week at the request of the attending (because of workload and team size). Sometimes no attending came to the rounding room, and I was unable to conduct observations.[11] After the first year of fieldwork, I would stay in the field for a few months and then step out to conduct preliminary data analysis. After completing the bulk of my research in August 2013, I returned to the field in the summer of 2015 for follow-up observations and interviews.

Over the course of a year, I also observed five IM hospitalist meetings dedicated to improving consultations. Each meeting began with a specialist presentation. Topics included general experiences consulting with the Internal Medicine service, problematic cases, and recommendations for improvement. An open discussion between IM and specialty physicians followed, where questions were asked and issues raised. Discussions ranged from thirty minutes to an hour. The meetings I attended were with Endocrinology, Gastroenterology, Pulmonology, Cardiology, and Rheumatology. There was a sixth meeting, with Infectious Disease, that I was unable to attend because I had not been notified of it.

Lastly, over the course of the study period I interviewed forty IM attending physicians and twenty-one IM trainees for a total of sixty-one interviews. Of the forty attendings, thirty-three were hospitalists and seven were internists.[12] Of the trainees, thirteen were second- or third-year residents, six were interns, one was a pediatric intern and internal medicine resident, and one was an ER resident. The interviews were conducted at a location of the interviewee's choosing. The attendings' interviews generally took place in their office or in a hospital meeting room. The trainees' interviews took place in the hospital cafeteria, in local restaurants or cafes near the hospital, in hospital lobbies, and in one case via video-chat. The interviews were audio-recorded (unless the interviewee refused consent) and fully transcribed. Interviews ranged from approximately twenty minutes to two hours.

As shown by the disparate numbers, it was very difficult to secure interviews with trainees largely because they did not respond to numerous personal emails. For those who did agree to be interviewed, I offered to buy a meal in exchange for their time. This allowed them to meet with me during their lunch break rather than taking time outside their busy work schedule. Nonetheless, even with meal offerings it remained very difficult to secure interviews. One explanation may be that trainees had less time than attendings. The difficulties I encountered may also reflect issues with social access that I will speak to next.

Notably missing here are formal interviews with case managers, nurses, and other medical staff. These individuals are undeniably critical to care delivery; however, I was unable to gain access to them. Only five case managers were assigned to the Internal Medicine Service, so they reported being too busy for interviews. The nurses were also inaccessible. Including them in my research would have required a separate hospital research review process, which would have taken too long for this study. I contacted several social workers, but none responded. The perceptions of nonphysician professionals would have enriched this book. Nevertheless, the hidden curriculum of doctoring and the lessons learned from it emerged clearly through my IM team observations and interviews.

UNEQUAL ACCESS IN THE FIELD

I experienced little difficulty fitting in with the IM teams during their morning rounds, as they were accustomed to unfamiliar persons such as trainees in other fields (e.g., nursing, pharmacy) and external researchers studying hospital efficiency and care delivery. Thus I became just one more team member.[13] Furthermore, as many team members jotted down notes during rounds, it was very easy for me to write my own unobtrusively.[14] Using a strategy adopted by many ethnographers, I offered to share my notes whenever anyone expressed interest or concern regarding my note-taking.

Social access was much more difficult to achieve uniformly across study participants.[15] Because I regularly attended morning rounds, the attendings and trainees began to recognize me and became friendlier. The attendings especially embraced my presence on the wards, which may have been a consequence of the IM director's interest in my work and his strong urging of his colleagues to participate. Many attendings took me under their wing. Perhaps as a student myself at the time, they saw me as another trainee to be mentored and supervised. They were patient and included me as much as possible during rounds, frequently asking if I had any questions, providing additional information, and explaining when I misunderstood something. Many also stayed behind after the team had dispersed to answer questions.

The trainees, on the other hand, were a much more closed network. Like other ethnographers,[16] I found it difficult to achieve meaningful relationships with the housestaff during morning rounds. I cannot be certain why, but I can draw some possible explanations from the scholarship. First, trainees may have seen me as aligned with supervisors since the attendings were my point of entry to the research site. Knee deep in clinical work and focused on their training, they may have felt that I had little to offer them. Some of my interviews with novice attendings supported this explanation, as many said that, because they were so overworked and tired, financial and social dimensions of care delivery were not on their minds during residency training. Only as attendings did they begin to think about "nonclinical" issues more seriously. Notably, however, some trainees were deeply invested in the financial, social, and bureaucratic dimensions of care delivery and concerned about the current structuring of the health care system and its effects on patient health and well-being. They stood out in their navigation of the hidden curriculum of doctoring, as their comments in interviews showed.

I had hoped to speak to many more trainees, but I do not believe the lack of interviews diminishes the story of the hidden curriculum; rather, it is a finding in and of itself. The inability to convince trainees to engage more deeply in this research may reveal both the importance of the health logic and the consequences of the training logic: clinical care and knowledge are privileged above all else at this point in trainees' careers. Furthermore, my observations of the IM teams and the informal conversations I had with them during morning rounds provided a clear picture of the struggles trainees undergo. In addition, many of the key lessons of the curriculum continue beyond residency, with some of the most critical lessons learned once trainees become attendings. Lastly, an interview sample that represents more attendings than trainings is not necessarily problematic.

ETHICAL CONCERNS IN THE FIELD

Research of any kind raises critical issues of ethics—informed consent, participants' privacy and confidentiality, the impact of findings on marginalized communities, among others—and my experience was no different. First, like other ethnographers,[17] I found it incredibly difficult, and sometimes impossible, to obtain informed consent from the consulting physicians, family members, nurse practitioners, social workers, hospital administrators, and other parties I encountered. Morning rounds tended to be unpredictable, with impromptu meetings between the IM team and colleagues taking place in hallways. In these interactions, I had no opportunity to request informed consent—unless I completely disrupted the conversation, which felt uncomfortable and inappropriate.[18] Rarely was my presence questioned because I blended in with the medical team. Fortunately, in more organized settings such as meetings and official consultations, the attending introduced me as a sociologist conducting research on the IM wards.

I experienced the tension between my desire to observe and my concerns about ethics most when dealing with patients and family members. While I had IRB approval to enter patient rooms, I let my access to these spaces be determined by the attending (some preferred I not enter), the team size (when teams were too large, I did not enter), and the patient and family.[19] In some instances, the attending failed to announce my presence. I felt uncomfortable because the patient and family were not aware of my purpose and because I was unable to identify myself. Over time some attendings announced me and asked the patient and family if they were comfortable with me in the room; other attendings did not, and in these cases I stayed in the hall.

Another ethical concern I grappled with was my intrusion into harrowing moments of patients' and families' lives. I observed patients crying as they received poor diagnoses and families struggling with the decision to transition their loved ones to hospice care. In acutely sensitive cases, the attending physician would notify me that difficult news was to be delivered and I stayed outside. In some cases, the family allowed my presence when meetings took place outside the patient's room and if they were alerted. I never took notes during these interactions

FINAL THOUGHTS

Ethnographers share the feeling that being in the field is incredibly complicated. We see the exciting, novel research emerging from our observations and fieldnotes but also recognize that our "findings" are real people, relationships, joys, and hardships. The hospital especially is a setting where ethnographic observations can seem inappropriate and cruel as patients and families face uncertainty and mortality. Understanding this, to the physicians, nurses, case managers, patients, families, and everyone else who allowed me a glimpse into their professional and personal worlds, I am forever grateful.

Glossary

Academic medical center: hospital affiliated with a medical school, administering clinical care, producing research, and providing clinical education for physicians-in-training.

Accreditation Council for Graduate Medical Education (ACGME): Organization that evaluates graduate medical training programs in the United States.

Afternoon interdisciplinary rounds: Meetings with the attending physician, resident, case manager, social worker, and other relevant staff. Unlike morning rounds, these last no more than thirty minutes, with the group quickly running through each patient and discussing social and financial issues related to patient care, particularly potential obstacles to discharge.

Almshouse: residence built and maintained by charitable individuals or organizations to house the poor, old, and ill.

Arterial blood gas (ABG) test: test to measure oxygen and carbon dioxide, as well as pH, in blood.

Attending physician: physician who provides care in the clinical setting and oversees the training and practice of medical students, interns, residents, and fellows.

Case manager: staff member who oversees patient care from a social and financial perspective and liaises with medical teams to ensure that social, financial, or organizational obstacles to care are avoided or quickly managed.

Centers for Medicare and Medicaid Services (CMS): federal agency in the Department of Health and Human Services that administers Medicare; with state governments, oversees Medicaid and the Children's Health Insurance Program (CHIP); and researches and evaluates various aspects of the US health care system.

Clinic: an outpatient clinical setting where usually hospital- or medical center–physicians see patients.

Colorectal: specialty service focused on conditions of the colon and rectum.

Computerized tomography (CT): imaging that combines x-rays taken at different angles to create cross-sections of the body

Consultant: specialist who, at the request of a primary care team, consults on a patient.

Crohn's disease: inflammatory bowel disease that affects the lining of the digestive tract.

Dermatology: specialty service focused on conditions of the skin.

Diagnosis-related group (DRG): patient classification scheme created in the 1970s to standardize hospital payments.

Differential diagnosis: determination of a particular disease or condition from a set of diseases or conditions that have similar symptoms.

Discharge: release of a patient from the hospital after an inpatient stay.

Discharge planner: staff member responsible for the release of a patient from the hospital to a safe place with access to necessary follow-up care.

Echocardiogram (Echo): sonogram imaging of the heart and valves.

Endocrinology: specialty service focused on conditions of the endocrine glands and hormones.

Fellowship: training period following the final year of residency.

Follow-up care: care received after hospital discharge, typically provided in an outpatient setting.

Gastroenterology (GI): specialty service focused on conditions of the gastrointestinal tract and liver.

Gynecology: specialty service focused on women's health, especially conditions of the reproductive system.

Hematology (Hem): specialty service focused on conditions of the blood

Hematology-Oncology (Hem-Onc): specialty service focused on diseases and cancers of the blood.

Home health: Skilled medical care provided in the home.

Hospice: Care provided to the terminally ill, specifically to make the patient as comfortable as possible either in a specialized facility or in the home.

Hospitalist: physician who works exclusively in the inpatient setting.

Housestaff: trainees in teaching hospitals, specifically interns and residents.

Inpatient care: care provided in the hospital.

Intern: first-year resident.

Interspecialty care: care incorporating multiple specialties.

Interventional radiology (IR): imaging of the body to diagnose injury or illness.

Intravenous therapy (IV): delivery of fluids directly into a vein.

Level I trauma center: tertiary care facility for all aspects of injury—from prevention through rehabilitation.

Lymphoma: cancer of the lymphocytes, infection-fighting cells that include lymph nodes, spleen, thymus, and bone marrow.

Magnetic resonance imaging (MRI): medical imaging that utilizes high-frequency radio waves to produce images of the internal organs.

Medicaid: public health insurance program that provides coverage to low-income families and to families and to individuals in one of the following categories: children, pregnant women, individuals over the age of 65, and individuals living with disabilities

Medi-Cal: State of California Medicaid program.

Medical specialization: Categories of medicine each of which focuses on a condition or group of conditions, organ group, procedure, and so forth.

Medicare: federal health insurance program for individuals 65 years of age or older.

Morning report: meeting of interns and residents to discuss interesting cases encountered on the wards.

Neurology (Neuro): specialty service focused on conditions of the nervous system.

Nursing home: facility that offers care to the elderly or the disabled.

Observation unit: hospital department that oversees patients who require medical monitoring and care but are not officially admitted to the hospital.

On call: care provided by a medical team overnight.

Ophthalmology: specialty service focused on conditions of the eye.

Out of pocket: costs of care for which the patient is responsible.

Outpatient care: care provided outside the hospital setting (e.g., clinic).

Palliative Care: specialty service that provides comfort care to seriously ill patients. Similar to hospice care but provided while the patient is receiving active treatment for an illness.

Patient-centered care: care delivery model that emphasizes patient involvement in care plans and medical decision-making.

Patient Protections and Affordable Care Act (ACA): federal law designed to make health coverage more equitable and accessible, to improve quality of care, and to reduce medical waste and unnecessary spending.

PO: orally/by mouth.

Positron emission tomography (PET): imaging using dye.

Postcall rounds: rounds completed after a team has worked overnight.

Primary care physician (PCP): physician who practices general medicine and is typically a patient's first stop for medical care.

Primary care team: medical team designated as medically and legally responsible for a patient's care.

Pulmonary/Pulmonology (Pulm): specialty service focused on conditions of the respiratory tract.

Quality improvement organization: organization of health quality experts, clinicians, and consumers established to improve the quality of care received by Medicare patients.

Radiology: medical imaging service.

Renal transplant: specialty service focused on kidney transplantation.

Residency: clinical training after medical school during which graduates select a specialty and, depending on the specialty, typically lasts three to seven years.

Resident: Medical trainee in a residency program.

Rheumatology (Rheum): specialty service that focuses on rheumatic conditions, which involve inflammation and pain in the joints, muscles, or fibrous tissue.

Senior resident: trainee in the final year of residency—the third year in Internal Medicine.

Skilled nursing facility (SNF, pronounced "sniff"): facility caring for hospital-discharged patients, usually temporarily, who require additional medical treatment.

Teaching hospital: health care center that provides medical education to future health care professionals.

Trainee: medical student or resident.

Transesophageal echocardiography (TEE): detailed imaging of the heart and arteries.

Urgent care: outpatient setting providing acute care.

Ward: hospital department or service.

Notes

CHAPTER 1

1. Cain 2019.

2. Studdert et al. 2000.

3. Chambliss 1996; Diamond 1992; Folbre 2012.

4. Kaufman 2005; Timmermans 1999.

5. The hidden curriculum refers to an informal, yet vital, training component that frequently emerges alongside formal education (Hafferty and Castellani 2009).

6. Beisecker and Beisecker, 1993; Emanuel and Emanuel 1992; Parsons 1951.

7. Freidson 1970b.

8. Greenwood and Lachman 1996; Reed 1996.

9. Conrad and Leiter 2004; Fennell and Alexander 1993; Light 2000.

10. Casalino 2004; Charles-Jones, Latimer, and May 2003.

11. Mechanic 1996.

12. Grumbach Osmond, Vranizan, Jaffe, and Bindman 1998; Kletke, Emmons, and Gillis 1996; Light 2000; Waitzkin 2000.

13. Patient-centered care is "respectful of and representative to individual patient preferences, needs, and values and ensuring that patient values guide all clinical decisions" (Committee on Quality of Health Care in America 2001:40).

14. Dunn and Jones 2010; Meyer et al. 1987; Thornton and Ocasio 1999, 2012.

15. D'Aunno et al. 1991; Friedland and Alford 1991; Greenwood et al. 2010; Meyer and Rowan 1977.

16. Besharov and Smith developed a framework to theorize how hybrid organizations work, arguing that their institutional outcome is contingent on the compatibility of the various logics present: Do these logics directly conflict with what they are prescribing or do they align? Another vital component is the centrality of these logics within the institution: Do they have equal weight in terms of the organization's primary objectives and goals? In some organizations with high incompatibility of institutional logics, there is a tendency to adopt isolated strategies and practices, where actor groups are differentiated based on their responsibility to meet the objectives of specific, conflicting institutional demands. This is particularly common in institutions where numerous member groups have distinct expertise and training. In other organizations, members absorb multiple logics at the same time, leading to integration rather than differentiation. Such organizations have multiple logics associated with high centrality—each one shapes daily work activities. Across these different organizational forms, there are generally three outcomes: one logic prevails above all others (the others remain in name only), "intractable conflict" emerges (deeply impinging on the organization's functioning), and "productive tension," where the various institutional logics coexist (Besharov and Smith 2014).

17. Troyer 2004.

18. DiMaggio 1997; Ocasio 1998; Thornton 2004.

19. Besharov and Smith 2014.

20. Battilana, Besharov and Mitzinneck 2017.

21. Battilana, Besharov and Mitzinneck 2017.

22. This is particularly common in institutions with numerous member groups with distinct expertise and training.

23. McPherson and Sauder 2013; Voronov, De Clercq, and Hinings 2013.

24. Dunn and Jones 2010; Lawrence, Suddaby, and Leca 2009; Martin et al. 2015.

25. Granovetter 1985; Rossman 2014; Zelizer 2005.

26. Zelizer 1979.

27. Almeling 2007; Livne 2014; Reich 2014; Zelizer 1979.

28. Altomonte 2020; Anteby 2010; Bandelj 2009.

29. Binder 2007; Cain 2019; McPherson and Sauder 2013.

30. Altomonte 2020:77.

31. Cain 2019.

32. Wennberg et al. 2008.

33. Smith Jr., Stein, and Jones 2012.

34. Hauer and Wachter 2001.

35. Wells et al. 2006.

36. Mickan 2005.

37. Solheim, McElmurry, and Kim 2007.

38. Wells et al. 2006.

39. Herrman, Trauer, and Warnock 2002.

40. Sands, Stafford, and McClelland 1990.

41. Finn, Learmonth, and Reedy 2010.

42. Leicht and Fennell 2001; Nancarrow and Borthwick 2005.

43. Starr 1982:356.

44. Abbott 1981; Leicht and Fennell 2001; Nancarrow and Borthwick 2005; Rosoff and Leone 1991.

45. Abbott 1981; Rosoff and Leone 1991.

46. Abbott 1981:823.

47. Liu and Kelz 2018.

48. Liu and Kelz 2018.

49. Cooke et al. 2006:n.p.

50. Though it should also be noted that trainees can financially benefit hospitals because interns and residents provide the bulk of daily care to further their medical education with minimal financial compensation.

51. University of Michigan n.d.

52. Pinsky 2000.

53. Fleishon et al. 2017:46.

54. The American Trauma Society defines a level-1 trauma center as "a comprehensive regional resource that is a tertiary care facility central to the trauma system . . . capable of providing total care for every aspect of injury—from prevention through rehabilitation."

55. Fisher 2019.

56. As physicians learn to provide care to uninsured and underinsured patients, they face the stark contradictions between the health and market logics.

57. Association of American Medical Colleges 2019.

58. In *Selling Our Souls: The Commodification of Hospital Care in the United States* (2014), Reich examines the impact of the commodification of care at three hospitals in the western United States: PubliCare, a hospital that historically has treated the underresourced; HolyCare, a hospital that was founded by an order of nuns; and GroupCare, an institution that serves primarily middle-class patients and their employers. He finds that the commodification of care, and its associated bureaucratization and cost-cutting initiatives, takes on divergent meanings and in turn diverse practices and policies at these institutions—shaping health care professionals' experiences, including their inter- and intraprofessional interactions, their relationships with patients, and even their compensation and

benefits. Notably absent in this study is an examination of academic medical centers, which Reich specifically addresses. He states that the academic medical center is "in many ways the heart of modern medical care, particularly in large metropolitan areas" (2014:195), alluding to the importance of studying the dynamics that arise in major teaching hospitals.

59. Fleishon et al. 2017:46.

60. Leicht and Fennell 1997.

61. Jenkins 2020.

62. Pearl 2017.

63. The Organization for Economic Co-operation and Development comprising 38 developed and developing countries that promotes global economic growth and trade.

64. Centers for Medicare and Medicaid Services 2018; OECD 2018.

65. OECD 2013.

66. Gibson and Waldo 1981.

67. Centers for Medicare and Medicaid 2014; 2018.

68. Wennberg, Fisher, Goodman, and Skinner 2008.

69. Wennberg et al. 2008.

CHAPTER 2

1. As noted in Chapter 1, while research logics are important in academic medical centers, they are not treated in this book because, in my experience, they were not an everyday concern for IM physicians on the clinical wards.

2. Trainees in their third year are referred to as residents or senior residents.

3. ACGME 2018:3–4.

4. Starr 1982.

5. A home for the poor, typically established by an individual or organization.

6. Starr 1982.

7. Johns Hopkins Medicine n.d.

8. Starr 1982.

9. de Luise 2014:3.

10. Epstein et al. 2010:1490.

11. Kupfer and Bond 2012:139.

12. Oshima, Emanuel, and Emanuel 2013.

13. Lyu et al. 2013.

14. Rothberg et al. 2014.

15. Mello et al. 2004.

16. Antoci, Maccioni, and Russu 2016; Sanger-Katz 2018; Vento, Cainelli, and Vallone 2018.

17. Eliot Freidson (1970b) has referred to professional dominance as the distinguishing trait of all professions. According to Freidson (1970b:xv), a "profession has assumed a dominant position in a division of labor, so that it gains control over the substance of its own work. Unlike most occupations, a profession is autonomous or self-directing and sustains this special status by its persuasive claim of the extraordinary trustworthiness of its members, which naturally includes ethicality and knowledgeable skill. In fact, the profession claims to be the most reliable authority on the reality it deals with. When it deals with the problems people bring to it, the profession develops an independent conception of those problems and tries to manage both client and problems in its own way."

18. Starr 1982.

19. Mechanic 1996.

20. In the early twentieth century, the doctor-patient relationship was characterized by medical paternalism, where the "general practitioner genuinely wants the best for the patient, but believes that patients often need to be guided firmly through the decision making process as they do not always know what is best for them" (McKinstry 1992:340). Paternalism was prominent during this time because of the identities accepted by patients and doctors. According to Talcott Parsons, patients assumed the "sick role," meaning "in a state where he is suffering or disabled or both, and possibly facing risks of worsening, which is socially defined as either not his fault or something from which he cannot be expected to extricate himself by his own effort, or generally both"(Parsons 1951:440). Furthermore, the patient "is not, of course competent to help himself" and so must seek "professional, technically competent help" (441). In this context, patients were not responsible for becoming ill but were responsible for seeking medical professionals in order to recover. They could not make any determinations regarding their health and well-being and instead had to place their full trust in the medical authority of physicians, granting them complete autonomy and control over all health care decisions (Reeder 1972).

21. Mangione-Smith, McGlynn, Elliott, Krogstad, and Brook 1999.

22. Catino 2011.

23. Mello et al. 2004.

24. Bone infection.

25. Patients' desire to remain in the hospital is not due solely to hospital amenities but are shaped by fear and knowledge of personal conditions and experiences outside the hospital.

26. Burns, Cacciamani, Clement, and Aquino 2000.

27. Burns et al. 2000.

28. Abelson 2009; Sanger-Katz 2018.

29. Healy 2019.

30. Healy 2019:n.p.

31. Abelson 2009.

32. Healy 2019.

33. Abelson 2018.

34. Beardwood, Walters, Eyles, and French 1999; Scott, Ruef, Mendel, and Caronna 2000.

35. Correia 2013; Martin et al. 2015; Scott et al. 2000.

36. Learmonth 1997.

37. Mechanic and McAlpine 2010.

38. Mechanic 2006.

39. Fisher et al. 2007.

40. Casalino 2004; Shortell and Casalino 2008.

41. Berwick and Hackbarth 2012.

42. Berwick and Hackbarth 2012.

43. Shrank, Rogstad, and Parekh 2019.

44. Originally the National Association of Inpatient Physicians, the only medical organization dedicated to hospitalists and hospital medicine.

45. Society of Hospital Medicine 2011.

46. Sox 1999.

47. Wachter 1999.

48. Bellet and Whitaker 2000; Palmer Jr. et al. 2001; Wachter and Goldman 2002.

49. Holliman, Dziegielewsk, and Datta 2001.

50. Holliman, et al. 2001.

51. Bellet and Whitaker 2000; Palmer Jr. et al. 2001; Wachter and Goldman 2002.

52. Gibson and Waldo 1981.

53. Centers for Medicare and Medicaid Services 2018.

54. Silbersweig 2016.

55. Roberts 2012.

56. Bosk 1979.

57. Mylotte, Kahler, and McCann 2001; Rosenthal et al. 1997.

58. Mechanic, Coleman, and Dobson 1998.

59. Khaliq et al. 2007.

60. Hauer et al. 2004.

61. Magee, Shields, and Nothnagle 2013.

62. Silbersweig 2016.

CHAPTER 3

1. Altomonte 2020:96.

2. Berg 1997; Berg and Bowker 1997; Heath 1982.

3. Pirkle, Dumont, and Zunzunegui 2012:564.

4. Romm and Putnam 1981:310.

5. Fisher and Shortell 2010; Greenhalgh, Potts, Wong, Bark, and Swingle-hurst 2009.

6. Adams, Mann, and Bauchner 2003; Glavan et al. 2008.

7. Bentley et al. 2008.

8. Institute of Medicine 2013.

9. A justifiable hospital stay is one deemed medically necessary and covered by the patient's insurer.

10. A surgical procedure to remove the spleen.

11. Shurtz 2013.

12. Abbott 1981; Hugman 1991.

13. Hanscom 2008.

14. Hartley 2002.

15. Gorman 2006.

16. Gorman 2006.

17. Prepaid physician services plans first appeared in 1939 in California. Eventually, Blue Cross and Blue Shield merged into the comprehensive health insurance plan that we know today.

18. Private insurance companies offered major medical insurance plans with significantly higher limits of coverage for catastrophic costs than Blue Cross, and included coverage for diagnostic tests, outpatient procedures, and doctors' visits. There was no coverage, however, for preventative services and primary and long-term care (Hoffman 2006).

19. This phenomenon is referred to as moral hazard, a concern still prominent in the current health care and health insurance landscape.

20. In the 1970s, the federal government intervened with legislation giving states the right to impose certificate of need laws. These laws enabled states to prohibit private acquisition of expensive medical technologies such as MRI machines, and blocked the construction of private hospitals.

21. Gorman 2006.

22. HMOs and PPOs are the predominant models of managed care.

23. Hoy, Curtis, and Rice 1991:19.

24. Wallack 1992:28.

25. Quadagno 2008.

26. Hafferty and Light 1995.

27. Mechanic 1996.

28. Mechanic 1996.

29. Mechanic 2008.

30. Popovic 2001.

31. Weiss and Elixhauser 2014.

32. Green and Thomas 2008.

33. Becker and Geer 1958; Newton, Barber, Clardy, Cleveland, and Patricia 2008.

34. Casalino et al. 2009.

35. It should be noted that surgeons and other specialists are just as likely (some, such as OB-GYNs, more so) to face legal risk.

36. Berg 1996:501.

CHAPTER 4

1. Solheim, McElmurry, and Kim 2007.

2. Wells et al. 2006.

3. Abbott 1988.

4. Bucher and Stelling 1969.

5. Abbott 1988.

6. Subspecialties include adolescent medicine, allergy and immunology, cardiology, endocrinology, gastroenterology, geriatrics, hematology, infectious disease, nephrology, oncology, pulmonology, rheumatology, and sports medicine.

7. Zetka Jr. 2001.

8. Interspecialty care has become more expected with the help of technology, which allows consultations beyond the inpatient setting, for instance via telemedicine (Lupton 2013).

9. Some conditions are included in a previously agreed-on list between the specialty and Internal Medicine that require specific consultants to be called immediately. Many of these lists were created through a dialogue between IM hospitalists and specialty attendings during the monthly hospitalist meetings that I attended.

10. Recommendations range from additional medical tests to consultations with other services.

11. Fellows have completed their residency and are in fellowship training. Interns are in their first year of residency training.

12. TEE (transesophageal echocardiography) provides detailed images of the heart and arteries.

13. "Mets" is short for "metastases," malignant growths that have emerged beyond the primary cancer site.

14. PET (positron emission tomography) provides imaging with dye.

15. Kobayashi et al. 2006.

16. Abbott 1981.

17. Rounds taking place after the team has been on call admitting and caring for patients overnight on the IM wards.

18. Jauhar 2014.

19. Serra 2010:174.

20. Nancarrow and Borthwick 2005.

21. Abbott 1981:823.

22. Abbott 1981.

23. Although Hugman (1991) differentiates the "virtuosos" from the general caregivers by occupational and professional group, the same logic can be applied when comparing IM physicians, or generalists, with consulting specialists.

24. Finn et al. 2010; Sanders and Harrison 2008.

25. O'Malley and Reschovsky 2011; Sutfcliffe, Lewton, and Rosenthal 2004.

26. The hospitalists on the Internal Medicine Service at PMC held monthly meetings during my fieldwork. For a year, the meetings focused on improving consultations. They engaged physicians from different consulting services in conversation about key issues in and obstacles to smooth and effective inter-specialty care.

27. Herrman, Trauer, and Warnock 2002.

28. Mizrahi 1986; Szymczak and Bosk 2012.

CHAPTER 5

1. Rau 2012.

2. Lavizzo-Mourey 2013:3.

3. Goodman, Fisher, and Chang 2013.

4. Lavizzo-Mourey 2013:3.

5. Chow 2013.

6. Centers for Medicare and Medicaid Services 2015:n.p.

7. Centers for Medicare and Medicaid Services 2015:n.p.

8. Fletcher 2016:n.p.

9. Roberts 2012:n.p.

10. This changed over the course of my research: PMC now has partnerships with some local SNFs, in which a certain number of beds are allocated to PMC patients. This does not always guarantee a free bed, but it does facilitate the process.

11. McGrath 2015.

12. Manary et al. 2013.

13. Bernabeo and Holmboe 2013; Mast, Hall, and Roter 2008; Roter and Hall 2006; Street Jr. et al. 2009.

14. Ocloo 2010.

15. Allsop, Jones, and Baggott 2004.

16. Mechanic 1996; Ozawa and Sripad 2013.

17. Allsop, Jones, and Baggott 2004; Mast, Hall, and Roter 2008; Ocloo 2010; Street Jr. et al. 2009.

18. Quill, Arnold, and Back 2009.

19. Epstein and Gramling 2013.

20. Koenig 2011; Roter and Hall 2006.

21. Bloomfield and Park 2017; Cobos, Haskard-Zolnierek, and Howard 2015.

22. Epstein and Peters 2009; Lichtenstein and Slovic 2006.

CHAPTER 6

1. Studies have also found great variation in consultation rates for Medicare patients in hospitals throughout the United States, even when controlling for differences across patient populations. Hospital size and geographic location are more important factors in predicting rates than the patient's medical conditions (Stevens et al. 2015). When patients' conditions and evidence-based decision-making are not the driving factors behind calling a specialist, there is a greater likelihood of consultant misuse.

2. Jauhar 2014:n.p.

3. Terhune 2017.

4. Consultations are not always a financial drain. Sometimes they can save money. Studies have shown that, particularly for patients with poor prognoses, Palliative Care minimizes unnecessary medical workups and treatments for terminally ill patients (O'Connor et al. 2018).

5. Financial implications are not the only consequence. Unnecessary care can place patients at increased emotional and physical risk (Cassel and Guest 2012).

6. Light 2000.

7. Physicians frequently prescribe unwarranted treatments and medications (Kravitz et al. 2005), adding to unnecessary health care spending.

8. Robinson 1986.

9. Gray 1993, 1997.

10. Defensive medicine is not new; it emerged out of the current landscape of patient centered care, which is attributed to the growing distrust of physicians and medicine (Mechanic 1996). Gone was the era of paternalism and in its place was a much more informed patient-consumer unafraid to make demands and

take legal action if dissatisfied (Mangione-Smith, McGlynn, Elliott, Krogstad, and Brook 1999.

11. Polanyi 1957 [1944].

12. Zelizer 1979, 2005.

13. Parsons 1951.

14. More seasoned attendings reported no financial training in residency either, demonstrating a shift toward financial issues in residency training in the last five to ten years.

15. This strategy was not solely driven by cost-cutting pressures. Rather, for trainees, already so deeply overburdened, discharging a patient lightened their workloads and opened up learning opportunities with the admission of new patients.

16. Apker and Eggly 2004; Becker et al. 1976; Bosk 2003.

17. Becker et al. 1976; Bosk 1979; Fox 1979; Lempp 2009; Riska 2009.

18. Fox 1979; Hafferty 1988; MacLeod 2001.

19. Hafferty and Castellani 2009.

20. Becker et al. 1976; Bosk 1979.

21. MacLeod 2001.

22. Becker and Geer 1958; Fox 1979; Morley et al. 2013.

23. Becker et al. 1976; Hafferty 2009; Hafferty and O'Donnell 2014; Hafler et al. 2011; Michalec 2012; Underman and Hirshfield 2016.

24. Abbott 1988; Freidson 1970a, 1970b; Leicht and Fennell 2001.

25. Fox 1957; Fox 1979; Light 1979.

26. Bosk 1979.

27. Coombs 1978; Hafferty 1988.

28. MacLeod 2001; Wear et al. 2006.

29. In his ethnography of surgical residency, Charles Bosk (1979) demonstrated how error management socializes residents to learn the moral values, expectations, and responsibilities held in highest regard by the medical profession. Firsthand experience with autopsies (Coombs 1978; Hafferty 1988) and terminal patients (MacLeod 2001; Wear et al. 2006) teach novice physicians to restrain their emotional response to provide objective and empathetic care.

30. Mechanic and McAlpine 2010.

31. Some lessons cannot be fully learned by interns and residents because their position in training and career shields them from some of the key lessons of doctoring. Attending physicians face obstacles and encounters that are vital to the livelihood of the profession—such as fears of litigation and the social issues that directly affect patient-physician and physician-family interactions.

32. AMA 2018.

33. Beasley, McBride, and Mcdonald 2009; Greenwald et al. 2006.

34. Mumford 1970.

35. Fordyce et al. 2012; Hagopian et al. 2004.

36. Timmermans 2020.

37. Gengler 2014:346.

38. Gengler 2014:346.

39. Andreassen and Trondsen 2010; Hibbard and Cunningham 2008; Salander and Moynihan 2010; Shim 2010.

40. Gage-Bouchard 2017; Hibbard and Cunningham 2008.

41. Quadagno 2008.

42. Wennberg et al. 2008.

43. Goodman et al. 2013; Lavizzo-Mourey 2013.

44. Health care costs have risen at a slightly slower rate than in previous years because of the ACA. However, they continue in the wrong direction and their growth may be accelerated by efforts to overhaul the Affordable Care Act.

45. Timmermans and Berg 2003.

46. Dixon-Woods et al. 2011.

47. Kaufman 2015:247.

48. Kaufman 2015:247.

49. Becker et al. 1976.

50. Ainsworth et al. 1991.

51. From a sociological perspective, there is a critical flaw in the current cost-cutting initiatives dealing with discharge and readmission: it has simply been reduced to a numbers game. In line with the broader movement toward standardization in medical care in the United States (Timmermans and Berg 2003), evaluation and penalization of hospitals is contingent on data that reports average lengths of stay and readmissions for individual hospitals. Standardized care privileges scientific evidence, usually in the form of statistical data, to shape how care is administered. But data ignores the broader social context in which a series of decisions determines why a patient remains in, or leaves, a hospital (Dixon-Woods, et al. 2011).

52. Baugh et al. 2012.

53. Beresford 2011:41.

54. Caramenico 2011.

55. Healy 2019.

56. Roberts 2012:n.p.

57. Wheeler et al. 2016.

58. Snoey 2018:n.p.

59. Snoey 2018:n.p.

60. Snoey 2018:n.p.
61. Commonwealth Fund 2015.
62. Thorlby and Arora 2015.
63. Thorlby and Arora 2015.
64. Thorlby and Arora 2015.
65. Allin and Rudoler 2015.
66. Choosing Wisely Canada 2015.
67. Matsuda 2015.
68. Matsuda 2015.
69. Liu and Haseltine 2015.
70. Liu and Haseltine 2015.

APPENDIX

1. The ethnographic nature of this project allowed me to become immersed in the hospital setting, to observe routine interactions and encounters. Bringing together various forms of data (observations, interviews, documents, and the like) allows generation of new hypotheses and theories along with a thick description of daily life events, and gives rise to practical recommendations (Emerson, 2001). Ethnography is "particularly useful . . . because we come closest to the people who are being studied. We can tell policy experts the implications of their policy on other people. We can tell policy people what the people that we have studied need in the way of policy" (Becker et al., 2004:265).

2. Bosk 1979; Chambliss 1996; Mizrahi 1986; Timmermans 1999; Zussman 1992.

3. Hertz and Imber 1995; Thomas 1995.

4. Hertz and Imber 1995:viii.

5. Thomas 1995:4–5.

6. Social scientists especially trigger alarms because there is concern about research reaching the media (Casper 1998). Accordingly, elites often have many "well-established and effective mechanisms for excluding social scientists" (Cassell 1988:93).

7. Bosk explains: "Access is not a single event but a continuous one" (1979:194), requiring constant negotiation and renegotiation of the researcher's presence. In *Sudden Death and the Myth of CPR*, Timmermans (1999) recounts a nine-month negotiation for access to two Emergency Departments at different hospitals. Neither hospital was familiar with ethnographic research and had concerns (one was liability) about a social scientist's presence during resuscitative efforts (Timmermans 1999).

8. Terry Mizrahi, in a study of the socialization of IM physicians (1986),

reflected on his good luck: the IM chairman was interested in sociology, so convincing him of the merits of the research was not difficult.

9. After two years of data collection at PMC, I tried to gain access to a county facility affiliated with it. However after corresponding with IM physicians there, I was unsuccessful.

10. "PMC" is a pseudonym, and pseudonyms have been used for all individuals. I also modified locations to preserve anonymity, such as where the Internal Medicine Service is housed at PMC.

11. Sometimes the teams met in the Observation Unit, the Emergency Department, a different office, or on another floor. These meetings were coordinated by pages and I did not know the location unless the attending emailed me directly.

12. Internists are IM physicians who primarily practice in the outpatient setting.

13. Zussman 1992.

14. Mizrahi 1986; Zussman 1992.

15. Anspach 1993; Millman, 1977.

16. Anspach (1993), during her initial observations of a neonatal intensive care unit (NICU), felt that she was in a "closed society" because it was exceedingly difficult to build relationships and trust with the staff. Others have noted that even after successfully negotiating physical access, research subjects tended to interact with the sociologist with suspicion (Millman 1977). In his 1995 study of hematologists, Atkinson wrote that his access to them was immediate because a colleague had negotiated for him. In contrast, access to pathologists was very difficult, with the senior pathologist remaining distanced and failing to introduce him to his colleagues. In his study of resuscitative efforts, even after receiving official access, Timmermans (1999) chose to volunteer at one of the hospitals to facilitate social access. This gave him opportunities to foster friendships with staff members. Heimer and Staffen (1998) also wrote about the difficulties of gaining social access in the NICU, emphasizing the numerous times they were asked, "Who are *you*?" which they translated as "Do you have a right to be here?" (378).

17. Bosk 1992; Diamond 1992.

18. Researchers must have a sense of when their presence is appropriate and when it is not (Cassell 1988); they must know and respect the limits of the studied group at different times and act according to the dynamics and situation at hand.

19. When patients were extremely sick and quarantined, I did not enter their rooms. Nor did I enter any patient's room when family did not want me. In some cases, however, physicians preferred my presence when dealing with patients with highly demanding family members.

Bibliography

Abbott, Andrew. 1981. "Status and Status Strain in the Professions." *American Journal of Sociology* 86(4):819–35.

Abbott, Andrew. 1988. *The System of Professions: An Essay on the Divison of Expert Labor.* Chicago: University of Chicago Press.

Abelson, Reed. 2009. "Insured, But Bankrupted by Health Crises." *New York Times*, June 30.

Abelson, Reed. 2018. "When Hospitals Merge to Save Money, Patients Often Pay More." *New York Times*, November 14.

Accreditation Council for Graduate Medical Education (ACGME). 2018. *ACGME Program Requirements for Graduate Medical Education in Internal Medicine.* Chicago: ACGME.

Adams, William G., Adriana M. Mann, and Howard Bauchner. 2003. "Use of an Electronic Medical Record Improves the Quality of Urban Pediatric Primary Care." *Pediatrics* 111(3):626–32.

Ainsworth, Michael A. et al. 1991. "Standardized Patient Encounters: A Method for Teaching and Evaluation." *JAMA* 266(10):1390–6.

Allin, Sara, and David Rudoler. 2015. "The Canadian Health Care System." *International Health Care System.* New York: Commonwealth Fund.

Allsop, Judith, Kathryn Jones, and Rob Baggott. 2004. "Health Consumer Groups in the UK: A New Social Movement?" *Sociology of Health and Illness* 26(6):737–56.

Almeling, Rene. 2007. "Selling Genes, Selling Gender: Egg Agencies, Sperm Banks, and the Medical Market in Genetic Material." *American Sociological Review* 72(3):319–40.

Altomonte, Guillermina. 2020. "Exploiting Ambiguity: A Moral Polysemy Approach to Variation in Economic Practices." *American Sociological Review* 85(1):76–105.

American Medical Association (AMA). 2018. "Freida Online®." Retrieved September 1, 2021 (http://www.ama-assn.org/ama/pub/education-careers/grad uate-medical-education/freida-online.page).

Andreassen, Hege, and Marianne Trondsen. 2010. "The empowered patient and the sociologist." *Social Theory and Health* 8(3):280–87.

Annandale, Ellen C. 1989. "The malpractice crisis and the doctor-patient relationship." *Sociology of Health and Illness* 11(1):1–23.

Anspach, Renee R. 1993. *Deciding Who Lives: Fateful Choices in the Intensive-Care Nursery.* Berkeley, CA: University of California Press.

Anteby, Michel. 2010. "Markets, Morals, and Practices of Trade: Jurisdictional Disputes in the U.S. Commerce in Cadavers." *Administrative Science Quarterly* 55(4):606–38.

Antoci, Angelo, Alessandro Fiori Maccioni, and Paolo Russu. 2016. "The Ecology of Defensive Medicine and Malpractice Litigation." *PLOS One* 11(3):1–15.

Armstrong, David. 2014. "Actors, Patients and Agency: A Recent History." *Sociology of Health and Illness* 36(2):163–74.

Association of American Medical Colleges. 2019. "Statement for the Record Submitted by the Association of American Medical Colleges (AAMC) to the Energy and Commerce Subcommittee on Health "Investing in America's Health Care." Retrieved March 6, 2022 (https://www.aamc.org/media/12486/).

Atkinson, Paul. 1995. *Medical Talk and Medical Work: The Liturgy of the Clinic.* London: Sage Publications.

Ayanian, John Z., and Joel S. Weissman. 2002. "Teaching Hospitals and Quality of Care: A Review of the Literature." *Milbank Quarterly* 80(3):569–93.

Bandelj, Nina. 2009. "Emotions in Economic Action and Interaction." *Theory and Society* 38(4):347–66.

Barker, Kristin. 2008. "Electronic Support Groups, Patient-Consumers, and Medicalization: The Case of Contested Illness." *Journal of Health and Social Behavior* 49:20–36.

Barker, Kristin K., and Cirila E. Vasquez Guzman. 2015. "Pharmaceutical Direct-to-Consumer Advertising and US Hispanic Patient-Consumers." *Sociology of Health and Illness* 37(8):1337–51.

Battilana, Julie, Marya Besharov, and Bjoern Mitzinneck. 2017. "On Hybrids and Hybrid Organizing: A Review and Roadmap for Future Research." Pp. 128-62 in *The SAGE Handbook of Organizational Institutionalism*. Edited by R. Greenwood, C. Oliver, T. B. Lawrence, and R. E. Meyer. Los Angeles, CA: SAGE.

Baugh, Christopher W., Arjun K. Venkatesth, Joshua A. Hilton, Peter A. Samuel, Jeremiah D. Schuur, and J. Stephen Bohan. "Making Greater Use Of Dedicated Hospital Observation Units For Many Short-Stay Patients Could Save $3.1 Billion A Year." *Health Affairs* 31(10):2314-23.

Beardwood, Barbara, Vivienne Walters, John Eyles, and Susan French. 1999. "Complaints against Nurses: A Reflection of 'the New Managerialism' and Consumerism in Health Care?" *Social Science and Medicine* 48(3):363-74.

Beasley, Brent, Jennifer McBride, and Furman McDonald. 2009. "Hospitalist Involvement in Internal Medicine Residencies." *Journal of Hospital Medicine* 4(8):471-75.

Becker, Howard S., and Blanche Geer. 1958. "The Fate of Idealism in Medical School." *American Sociological Review* 23(1):50-6.

Becker, Howard S., Herbert J. Gans, Katherine S. Newman, and Diane Vaughan. 2004. "On the Value of Ethnography: Sociology and Public Policy: A Dialogue." *Annals of the American Academy of Political and Social Science* 595(1):264-76.

Becker, Howard S., Blanche Geer, Everett C. Hughes, and Anselm Strauss. 1976. *Boys in White: Student Culture in Medical School*. New Brunswick, NJ: Transaction Publications.

Beisecker, Analee E., and Thomas D. Beisecker. 1993. "Using Metaphors to Characterize Doctor-Patient Relationships: Paternalism versus Consumerism." *Health Communication* 5(1):41-58.

Bellet, Paul S., and Robert C. Whitaker. 2000. "Evaluation of a Pediatric Hospital Service: Impact on Length of Stay and Hospital Charges." *Pediatrics* 105(3):478-84.

Bentley, Tanya G. K., Rachel M. Effros, Kartika Palar, and Emmett B. Keeler. 2008. "Waste in the U.S. Health Care System: A Conceptual Framework." *Milbank Quarterly* 86(4):629-59.

Beresford, Larry. 2011. "Is a Post-discharge Clinic in Your Hospital's Future?" *Hospitalist,* 15(12):41-2.

Berg, Marc. 1996. "Practices of Reading and Writing: The Constitutive Role of the Patient Record in Medical Work." *Sociology of Health and Illness* 18(4):499-524.

Berg, Marc. 1997. "Of Forms, Containers, and the Electronic Medical Record: Some Tools for a Sociology of the Formal." *Science, Technology, and Human Values* 22(4):403–33.

Berg, Marc, and Geoffrey Bowker. 1997. "The Multiple Bodies of the Medical Record: Toward a Sociology of an Artifact." *Sociological Quarterly* 38(3):513–37.

Bergen, Clara, Tanya Stivers, Rebecca K. Barnes, John Heritage, Rose McCabe, Laura Thompson, and Merran Toerrien. 2017. "Closing the Deal: A Cross-Cultural Comparison of Treatment Resistance." *Health Communication* 33(11):1–12.

Bernabeo, Elizabeth, and Eric S. Holmboe. 2013. "Patients, Providers, and Systems Need to Acquire a Specific Set of Competencies to Achieve Truly Patient-Centered Care." *Health Affairs* 32(2): 250–58.

Berwick, Donald M., and Andrew D. Hackbarth. 2012. "Eliminating Waste in US Health Care." *JAMA* 307(14):1513–16.

Besharov, Marya, and Wendy K. Smith. 2014. "Multiple Institutional Logics in Organizations: Explaining Their Varied Nature and Implication." *Academy of Management Review* 39(3):364–81.

Binder, Amy. 2007. "For Love and Money: Organizations' Creative Responses to Multiple Environmental Logics." *Theory and Society* 36(6):547–71.

Bloomfield, Dennis A., and Alex Park. 2017. "Decoding White Coat Hypertension." *World Journal of Clinical Cases* 15(3):82–92.

Bosk, Charles L. 1979. *Forgive and Remember: Managing Medical Failure.* Chicago: University of Chicago Press.

Bosk, Charles L. 1992. *All God's Mistakes: Genetic Counseling in a Pediatric Hospital."* Chicago: University of Chicago Press.

Bucher, Rue, and Joan Stelling. 1969. "Characteristics of Professional Organizations." *Journal of Health and Social Behavior* 10(1):3–15.

Burns, Lawton R., John Cacciamani, James Clement, and Welman Aquino. 2000. "The Fall of the House of AHERF: The Allegheny Bankruptcy." *Health Affairs* 19(1):7–41.

Cain, Cindy L. 2019. "Agency and Change in Healthcare Organizations: Workers' Attempts to Navigate Multiple Logics in Hospice Care." *Journal of Health and Social Behavior* 60(1):3–17.

Caramenico, Alicia. 2011. "Hospitals Use Post-Discharge Clinics to Cut Readmissions." *FierceHealth care.* Retrieved April 29, 2014 (https://www.fiercehealth care .com/health care/hospitals-use-post-discharge-clinics-to-cut-readmissions).

Casalino, Lawrence P. 2004. "Unfamiliar Tasks, Contested Jurisdictions: The Changing Organization Field of Medical Practice in the United States." *Journal of Health and Social Behavior* 45(Supplement):59–75.

Casalino, Lawrence P., Sean Nicholson, David N. Gans, Terry Hammons, Dante Morra, Theodore Karrison, and Wendy Levinson. 2009. "What Does It Cost Physician Practices to Interact with Health Insurance Plans?" *Health Affairs* 28(1):web exclusive. Retrieved March 24, 2022 (https://www.healthaffairs.org/doi/10.1377/hlthaff.28.4.w533).

Casper, Monica J. 1998. *The Making of the Unborn Patient: A Social Anatomy of Fetal Surgery*. New Brunswick, NJ: Rutgers University Press.

Cassel, Christine K., and James A. Guest. 2012. "Choosing Wisely: Helping Physicians and Patients Make Smart Decisions About Their Care." *JAMA* 307(17):1801–02.

Cassell, Joan. 1988. "The Relationship of Observer to Observed When Studying Up." In *Studies in Qualitative Methodology: Conducting Qualitative Research*. Edited by R. G. Burgess, 89-108. Greenwich, CT: JAI Press Inc.

Catino, Maurizio. 2011. "Why Do Doctors Practice Defensive Medicine? The Side-Effects of Medical Litigation." *Safety Science Monitor* 15(1):1–12.

Centers for Medicare and Medicaid Services. 2014. NHE Fact Sheet. Baltimore, MD. Retrieved 4/25/2014

Centers for Medicare and Medicaid Services. 2015. "Discharge Planning Proposed Rule Focuses on Patient Preferences." Retrieved June 5, 2017 (https://www.cms.gov/newsroom/press-releases/discharge-planning-proposed-rule-focuses-patient-preferences).

Centers for Medicare and Medicaid Services. 2018. National Health Expenditures 2017 Highlights. Baltimore, MD: Centers for Medicare and Medicaid Services.

Chambliss, Daniel F. 1996. *Beyond Caring: Hospitals, Nurses, and the Social Organization of Ethics*. Chicago: University of Chicago Press.

Charles-Jones, Huw, Joanna Latimer, and Carl May. 2003. "Transforming General Practice: The Redistribution of Medical Work in Primary Care." *Sociology of Health and Illness* 25(1):71–92.

Choosing Wisely Canada. 2015. "Becoming a Choosing Wisely Canada Hospital." *ChoosingWiselyCanada.org*. Retrieved September 10, 2019 (https://choosingwiselycanada.org/campaign/hospitals/).

Chow, Lisa. 2013. "3 Ways Obamacare is Changing How a Hospital Cares for Patients." *NPR.org*. Retrieved October 10, 2018 (https://www.npr.org/sections/money/2013/12/02/247216805/three-ways-obamacare-is-changing-how-a-hospital-cares-for-patients).

Cobos, Briana, Kelly B. Haskard-Zolnierek, and Krista Howard. 2015. "White Coat Hypertension: Improving the Patient-Health Care Practitioner Relationship." *Psychology Research and Behavior Management* 8(May 2):133–41.

Committee on Quality of Health Care in America (Institute of Medicine). 2001. *Crossing the Quality Chasm: A New Health System for the 21st Century.* Washington, DC: National Academy Press.

Conrad, Peter, and Valerie Leiter. 2004. "Medicalization, Markets and Consumers." Extra issue, *Journal of Health and Social Behavior* 45:158–76.

Cooke, Molly, David M. Irby, William Sullivan, and Kenneth M. Ludmerer. 2006. "American Medical Education 100 Years after the Flexner Report." *New England Journal of Medicine* 355:1339–44.

Coombs, Robert H. 1978. *Mastering Medicine: Professional Socialization in Medical School.* New York: Free Press.

Correia, Tiago. 2013. "The Interplay between Managerialism and Medical Professionalism in Hospital Organisations from the Doctors' Perspective: A Comparison of Two Distinctive Medical Units." *Health Sociology Review* 22(3): 255–67.

D'Aunno, Thomas, Robert I. Sutton, and Richard H. Price. 1991 "Isomorphism and External Support in Conflicting Institutional Environments: A Study of Drug Abuse Treatment Units." *Academy of Management Journal* 34:636–61.

de Luise, Vincent P. 2014. "Teachable Moments, Learnable Moments: Medical Rounds as a Paradigm for Education." *Mind, Brain, and Education* 8(1):3–5.

Diamond, Timothy. 1992. *Making Gray Gold: Narratives of Nursing Home Care.* Chicago: University of Chicago Press.

DiMaggio, Paul J. 1997. "Culture and Cognition." *Annual Review of Sociology* 23(1):263–87.

Dixon-Woods, Mary, Charles L. Bosk, Emma-Louise Aveling, Christine A. Goeschel, and Peter J. Pronovost. 2011. "Explaining Michigan: Developing an Ex Post Theory of a Quality Improvement Program." *Milbank Quarterly* 89(2):167–205.

Dunn, Mary B., and Candace Jones. 2010. "Institutional Logics and Institutional Pluralism: The Contestation of Care and Science Logics in Medical Education, 1967–2005." *Administrative Science Quarterly* 55(1):114–49.

Eisenhardt, Kathleen M. 1989. "Building Theories from Case Study Research." *Academy of Management Review* 14(4):532–50.

Emanuel, Ezekiel J., and Linda L. Emanuel. 1992. "Four Models of the Physician-Patient Relationship." *Journal of the American Medical Association* 267:2221–26.

Emerson, Robert M. 2001. *Contemporary Field Research: Perspectives and Formulations.* Prospect Heights, IL: Waveland Press.

Epstein, Ronald M., and Robert E. Gramling. 2013. "What Is Shared in Shared Decision Making? Complex Decisions When the Evidence Is Unclear." Supplement, *Medical Care Research and Review* 70(1):94S-112S.

Epstein, Ronald M., and Ellen Peters. 2009. "Beyond Information: Exploring Patients' Preferences." *Journal of the American Medical Association* 302(2):195–97.

Epstein, Ronald M., Kevin Fiscella, Cara S. Lesser, and Kurt C. Stange. 2010. "Why the Nation Needs a Policy Push on Patient-Centered Health Care." *Health Affairs* 29(8):1489–95.

Exworthy, Mark, et al. 2003. "The role of performance indicators in changing autonomy of the general practice profession in the UK." *Social Science and Medicine* 56(7):1493–504.

Fennell, Mary L., and Jeffrey A. Alexander. 1993. "Perspectives on Organizational Change in the US Medical Care Sector." *Annual Review of Sociology* 19:89–112.

Fenton, Anny T. 2019. "Abandoning Medical Authority: When Medical Professionals Confront Stigmatized Adolescent Sex and the Human Papillomavirus (HPV) Vaccine." *Journal of Health and Social Behavior* 60(2):240–56.

Finn, Rachael, Mark Learmonth, and Patrick Reedy. 2010. "Some unintended effects of teamwork in health care." *Social Science & Medicine* 70(8):1148–54.

Fisher, Elliott S., and Stephen M. Shortell. 2010. "Accountable Care Organizations: Accountable for What, to Whom, and How." *JAMA* 304(15):1715–16.

Fisher, Elliott S., Douglas O. Staiger, Julie P. W. Bynum, and Daniel J. Gottlieb. 2007. "Creating Accountable Care Organizations: The Extended Hospital Medical Staff." *Health Affairs* 26(1):web exclusive. Retrieved March 24, 2022 (https://www.healthaffairs.org/doi/10.1377/hlthaff.26.1.w44).

Fisher, Karen. 2019. "Academic Health Centers Save Millions of Lives."*AAMC News and Insights*. Retrieved March 6, 2022 (https://www.aamc.org/news-insights/academic-health-centers-save-millions-lives).

Fleishon, Howard B., Jason N. Itri, Giles W. Boland, and Richard Duszak Jr. 2017. "Academic Medical Centers and Community Hospitals Integration: Trends and Strategies." *Journal of the American College of Radiology* 14:45–51.

Fletcher, Karen. 2016. "New California Law Involves Family Caregivers in Discharge Planning." *California Health Advocates*. Retrieved August 10, 2017 (https://cahealthadvocates.org/new-california-law-involves-family-caregivers-in-discharge-planning/).

Folbre, Nancy, ed. 2012. *For Love and Money: Care Provision in the United States.* New York: Russell Sage Foundation.

Fordyce, Meredith A., Mark P. Doescher, Frederick M. Chen, and L. Gary Hart. 2012. "Osteopathic Physicians and International Medical Graduates in the Rural Primary Care Physician Workforce." *Family Medicine* 44(6):396–403.

Fox, Renee C. 1957. "Training for Uncertainty." In *The Student-Physician*. Edited by R. K. Merton, G. Reader, and P. L. Kendall, 207–241. Cambridge, MA: Harvard University Press.

Fox, Renee C. 1979. *Essays in Medical Sociology: Journeys into the Field*. New York: John Wiley & Sons.

Friedland, Roger, and Robert R. Alford. 1991. "Bringing Society Back In: Symbols, Practices, and Institutional Contradictions." In *The New Institutionalism in Organizational Analysis*. Edited by W.W. Powell, and P. J. Dimaggio, 232–63. Chicago, IL: University of Chicago Press.

Freidson, Eliot. 1970. *Profession of Medicine: A Study of the Sociology of Applied Knowledge*. New York: Harper and Row.

Freidson, Eliot. 1970. *Professional Dominance: The Social Structure of Medical Care*. New York: Atherton Press.

Gage-Bouchard, Elizabeth A. 2017. "Culture, Styles of Institutional Interactions, and Inequalities in Healthcare Experiences." *Journal of Health and Social Behavior* 58(2):147–65.

Gengler, Amanda N. 2014. "'I Want You to Save My Kid!': Illness Management Strategies, Access, and Inequality at an Elite University Research Hospital." *Journal of Health and Social Behavior* 55(3):342–59.

Gibson, Robert M., and Daniel R. Waldo. 1981. "National Health Expenditures, 1980." *Health Care Financing Review* 3(1):1–54.

Glavan, Bradford J., Ruth A. Engelberg, Lois Downey, and J. Randall Curtis. 2008. "Using the Medical Record to Evaluate the Quality of End-of-Life Care in the Intensive Care Unit." *Critical Care Medicine* 36(4):1138–48.

Goodman, David C., Elliott S. Fisher, and Chiang-Hua Chang. 2013. "After Hospitalization: A Dartmouth Atlas Report on Readmissions among Medicare Beneficiaries." In *The Revolving Door: A Report on U.S. Hospital Readmissions*. Edited by Perry Undem Research and Communication, 7–30. Princeton, NJ: Robert Wood Johnson Foundation.

Gorman, Linda. 2006. *The History of Health Care Costs and Health Insurance*. Milwaukee: Wisconsin Policy Research Institute.

Granovetter, Mark. 1985. "Economic Action and Social Structure: The Problem of Embeddedness." *American Journal of Sociology* 191(3):481–510.

Gray, Bradford H. 1997. "Trust and Trustworthy Care in the Managed Care Era." *Health Affairs* 16(1):34–49.

Gray, Bradford H. 1993. *The Profit Motive and Patient Care: The Changing Accountability of Doctors and Hospitals.* Cambridge, MA: Harvard University Press.

Green, Shayla D., and Joan D. Thomas. 2008. "Interdisciplinary Collaboration and the Electronic Medical Record." *Pediatric Nursing* 34(3):225.

Greenhalgh, Trisha, Henry W. W. Potts, Geoff Wong, Pippa Bark, and Deborah Swinglehurst. 2009. "Tensions and Paradoxes in Electronic Patient Record Research: A Systematic Literature Review Using the Meta-Narrative Method." *Milbank Quarterly* 87(4):729–88.

Greenwald, Leslie, et al. 2006. "Specialty versus Community Hospitals: Referrals, Quality, and Community Benefits." *Health Affairs* 25(1):106–18.

Greenwood, Royston, and Ran Lachman. 1996. "Change as an Underlying Theme in Professional Service Organizations: An Introduction." *Organization Studies* 17(4):563–72.

Greenwood, Royston, Amalia Magán Díaz, Stan Xiao Li, and José Céspedes Lorente, 2010. "The Multiplicity of Institutional Logics and the Heterogeneity of Organizational Responses." *Organization Science* 21(2):521–39

Grumbach, Kevin, Dennis Osmond, Karen Vranizan, Deborah Jaffe, and Andrew B. Bindman. 1998. "Primary Care Physicians' Experience of Financial Incentives in Managed-Care Systems." *New England Journal of Medicine* 339:1516–21.

Hafferty, Frederic W. 1988. "Cadaver Stories and the Emotional Socialization of Medical Students." *Journal of Health and Social Behavior* 29():344–56.

Hafferty, Frederic W. 2009. "Professionalism and the Socialization of Medical Students." In *Teaching Medical Professionalism.* Edited by R. L. Cruess, S. R. Cruess, and Y. Steinert, 53–70. New York: Cambridge University Press.

Hafferty, Frederic W., and Brian Castellani. 2009. The Hidden Curriculum: A Theory of Medical Education. in *Handbook of the Sociology of Medical Education.* Edited by C. Brosnan and B. S. Turner, 15–35. London: Routledge.

Hafferty, Frederic W., and Joseph F. O'Donnell. 2014. *The Hidden Curriculum in Health Professional Education.* Lebanon, NH: Trustees of Dartmouth College.

Hafferty, Frederic W., and Donald W. Light. 1995. "Professional Dominance and the Changing Nature of Medical Work." Extra issue, *Journal of Health and Social Behavior* 35:132–53.

Hafler, Janet P, et al. 2011. Decoding the Learning Environment of Medical Education: A Hidden Curriculum Perspective for Faculty Development. *Academic Medicine* 86(4):440–44.

Hagopian, Amy, Matthew Thompson, Emily Kaltenbach, and L. Gary Hart. 2004. "The Role of International Medical Graduates in America's Small Rural Critical Access Hospitals." *Journal of Rural Health* 20(1):52–58.

Halpern, Sydney A. 2004. "Medical Authority and the Culture of Rights." *Journal of Health Politics, Policy and Law* 29(4–5):835–52.

Hanscom, Robert. 2008. "Medical Simulation from an Insurer's Perspective." *Academic Emergency Medicine* 15(11):984–87.

Hartley, Heather. 2002. "The System of Alignments Challenging Physician Professional Dominance: An Elaborated Theory of Countervailing Powers." *Sociology of Health and Illness* 24:178–207.

Hauer, Karen E., and Robert Wachter. 2001. "Implications of the Hospitalist Model for Medical Students' Education." *Academic Medicine: Journal of the Association of American Medical Colleges* 76(4):324–30.

Hauer, Karen E., Robert M. Wachter, Charles E. McCulloch, Garmen A. Woo, and Andrew D. Auerbach. 2004. "Effects of Hospitalist Attending Physicians on Trainee Satisfaction with Teaching and with Internal Medicine Rotations." *Archives of Internal Medicine* 164(17):1866-71.

Healy, Jack. 2019. "Nursing Homes Are Closing Across Rural America, Scattering Residents." *New York Times*, March 4. Retrieved March 24, 2022 (https://www.nytimes.com/2019/03/04/us/rural-nursing-homes-closure.html).

Heath, Christian. 1982. "Preserving the consultation: medical record cards and professional conduct." *Sociology of Health and Illness* 4(1):56–74.

Heimer, Carol A., and Lisa R. Staffen. 1998. *For the Sake of the Children: The Social Organization of Responsibility in the Hospital and the Home.* Chicago, IL: University of Chicago Press.

Herrman, Helen, Tom Trauer, Julie Warnock, and Professional Liaison Committee (Australia) Project Team. 2002. "The Roles and Relationships of Psychiatrists and Other Service Providers in Mental Health Services." *Australian and New Zealand Journal of Psychiatry* 36(1):75–80.

Hertz, Rosanna, and Jonathan B. Imber. 1995. "Introduction." In *Studying Elites Using Qualitative Methods.* Edited by R. Hertz and J. B. Imber, vii-xi. Thousand Oaks, CA: Sage.

Hibbard, Judith H., and Peter J. Cunningham. 2008. "How Engaged Are Consumers in Their Health and Health Care, and Why Does It Matter." *Research Brief* 8(October):1–9.

Hoffman, Sharona. 2006. "Employing E-Health: The Impact of Electronic Health Records on the Workplace." *Faculty Publications.* Cleveland, OH: Case Western University School of Law.

Holliman, Diane C., Sophia F. Dziegielewsk, and Priyadarshi Datta. 2001. "Discharge Planning and Social Work Practice." *Social Work in Health Care* 32(3):1–19.

Holton, Judith A. 2007. "The Coding Process and Its Challenges." In *The Sage Handbook of Grounded Theory*, edited by A. Bryant and K. Charmaz, 265–89. Los Angeles: SAGE.

Hoy, Elizabeth W., Richard E. Curtis, and Thomas Rice. 1991. "Change and Growth in Managed Care." *Health Affairs* 10(4):18–36.

Hugman, Richard. 1991. *Power in Caring Professions*. Houndsmill, UK: Macmillan.

Institute of Medicine. 2013. *Best Care at Lower Cost: The Path to Continuously Learning Health Care in America*. Washington, DC: National Academies Press.

Jauhar, Sandeep. 2014. "One Patient, Too Many Doctors: The Terrible Expense of Overspecialization." *Time*, August 19.

Jenkins, Tania M. 2018. "Dual Autonomies, Divergent Approaches: How Stratification in Medical Education Shapes Approaches to Patient Care." *Journal of Health and Social Behavior* 59(2): 268–82.

Jenkins, Tania. 2020. *Doctors' Orders: The Making of Status Hierarchies in an Elite Profession*. New York: Columbia University Press.

Johns Hopkins Medicine. n.d. *Who Was Johns Hopkins?* Baltimore, MD: Johns Hopkins Medicine Marking and Communications Office.

Kahn, Robert, Donald M. Wolfe, Robert P. Quinn, J. Diedrick Snoek, and Robert A. Rosenthal. 1964. *Organizational Stress: Studies in Role Conflict and Ambiguity*. New York: Wiley.

Kaufman, Sharon. 2005. *And a Time to Die: How American Hospitals Shape the End of Life*. Chicago: Chicago University Press.

Kaufman, Sharon. 2015. *Ordinary Medicine: Extraordinary Treatments, Longer Lives, and Where to Draw the Line*. Durham, NC: Duke University Press.

Kelle, Udo. 2007. "The Development of Categories: Different Approaches in Grounded Theory." In *The Sage Handbook of Grounded Theory*, edited by A. Bryant and K. Charmaz, 191–213. Los Angeles: Sage.

Kellogg, Katherine. 2011. *Challenging Operations: Medical Reform and Resistance in Surgery*. Chicago: Chicago University Press.

Khaliq, Amir A., Chiung-Yu Huang, Apar Kishor Ganti, and Kristie Invie. 2007. "Comparison of Resource Utilization and Clinical Outcomes between Teaching and Nonteaching Medical Services." *Journal of Hospital Medicine* 2(3):150-7.

Kletke, Phillip R., David W. Emmons, and Kurt D. Gillis. 1996. "Current Trends in Physicians' Practice Arrangements: From Owners to Employees." *JAMA* 276(7):555–60.

Kobayashi, H., May Pian-Smith, M. Sato, R. Sawa, Toshiyuki Takeshita, and D. Raemer. 2006. "A Cross-Cultural Survey of Residents' Perceived Barriers in Questioning/Challenging Authority." *Quality and Safety in Health Care* 15(4):277–83.

Koenig, Christopher J. 2011. "Patient Resistance as Agency in Treatment Decisions." *Social Science and Medicine* 72:1105–14.

Kravitz, Richard L., Ronald M. Epstein, Mitchell D. Feldman, Carol E. Franz, Azari Rahman, Michael S. Wilkes, Ladson Hinton, and Peter Franks. 2005. "Influence of Patients' Requests for Direct-to-Consumer Advertised Antidepressants: A Randomized Controlled Trial." *JAMA* 293:1995–2002.

Kupfer, Joel M., and Edward U. Bond. 2012. "Patient Satisfaction and Patient-Centered Care: Necessary But Not Equal." *JAMA* 308(2):139–40.

Lawrence, Thomas B., Roy Suddaby, and Bernard Leca, eds. 2009. *Institutional Work: Actors and Agency in Institutional Sudies of Organizations*. Cambridge, UK: Cambridge University Press.

Lavizzo-Mourey, Risa. 2013. Introduction to *The Revolving Door: A Report on U.S. Hospital Readmissions*, edited by Perry Undem Research and Communication, 3–6. Princeton, NJ: Robert Wood Johnson Foundation.

Learmonth, Mark. 1997. "Managerialism and Public Attitudes towards UK NHS Managers." *Journal of Management in Medicine* 11(4):214–21.

Leicht, Kevin T., and Mary L. Fennell. 1997. "The Changing Organizational Context of Professional Work." *Annual Review of Sociology* 23:215–31.

Leicht, Kevin T., and Mary L. Fennell. 2001. *Professional Work: A Sociological Approach*. Malden, MA: Blackwell.

Lempp, Heidi. 2009. Medical-School Culture. In *Handbook of the Sociology of Medical Education*, edited by C. Brosnan and B. S. Turner, 71–88. London: Routledge Taylor & Francis Group.

Lichtenstein, Sarah, and Paul Slovic. 2006. *The Construction of Preference*. Cambridge, UK: Cambridge University Press.

Light, Donald W. 1979. "Uncertainty and Control in Professional Training." *Journal of Health and Social Behavior* 20(4):310–22.

Light, Donald W. 2000. "The Medical Profession and Organizational Change: From Professional Dominance to Countervailing Power." In *Handbook of Medical Sociology*, vol. 5, edited by C. E. Bird, P. Conrad, and A. M. Fremont, 201–16. Upper Saddle River, NJ: Prentice Hall.

Light, Donald W., and Sol Levine. 1988. "The Changing Character of the Medical Profession: A Theoretical Overview." Supplement, *Milbank Quarterly* 66(2): S10–32.

Liu, Chang, and William Haseltine, 2015. "The Singaporean Health Care System." *International Health Care System*. New York: Commonwealth Fund.

Liu, Jason, and Rachel R. Kelz. 2018. "Types of Hospitals in the United States." *JAMA* 320(10):1074.

Livne, Roi. 2014. "Economies of Dying: The Moralization of Economic Scarcity in U.S. Hospice Care." *American Sociological Review* 79(5):888–911.

Lupton, Deborah. 2013. The digitally engaged patient: Self-monitoring and self-care in the digital health era." *Social Theory & Health* 11(3): 256–70.

Lyu, Heather, Elizabeth C. Wick, Michael Housman, Julie Ann Freischlag, and Martin A. Makary. 2013. "Patient Satisfaction as a Possible Indicator of Quality Surgical Care." *JAMA Surgery* 148(4):362–37.

MacLeod, Rod D. 2001. "On Reflection: Doctors Learning to Care for People Who Are Dying." *Social Science and Medicine* 52(11):1719–27.

Magee, Susanna R., Robin J. Shields, and Melissa B. Nothnagle. 2013. "Low Cost, High Yield: Simulation of Obstetric Emergencies for Family Medicine Training." *Teaching and Learning in Medicine* 3:207–10.

Manary, Matthew P., William Boulding, Richard Staelin, and Seth W. Glickman. 2013. "The Patient Experience and Health Outcomes." *New England Journal of Medicine* 368:201–03.

Mangione-Smith, Rita, Elizabeth A. McGlynn, Marc N. Elliott, Paul Krogstad, and Robert H. Brook. 1999. "The Relationship between Perceived Parental Expectations and Pediatrician Antimicrobial Prescribing Behavior." *Pediatrics* 103(4 pt. 1):711–18.

Mangione-Smith, Rita, Tanya Stivers, Marc N. Elliott, Laurie McDonald, and John Heritage. 2003. "Online Commentary during the Physical Examination: A Communication Tool for Avoiding Inappropriate Antibiotic Prescribing?" *Social Science and Medicine* 56(2):313–20.

Martin, Graham P., Natalie Armstrong, Emma-Louise Aveling, Georgia Herbert, and Mary Dixon-Woods. 2015. "Professionalism Redundant, Reshaped, or Reinvigorated? Realizing the "Third Logic" in Contemporary Health Care." *Journal of Health and Social Behavior* 56(3):378–97.

Mast, Marianne Schmid, Judith A. Hall, and Debra L. Roter. 2008. "Caring and Dominance Affect Participants' Perceptions and Behaviors During a Virtual Medical Visit." *Journal of General Internal Medicine* 23(5):523–27.

Matsuda, Ryozo. 2015. "The Japanese Health Care System." *International Health Care System*. New York: Commonwealth Fund.

McGrath, Dan. 2015. "There Aren't Enough Nursing-Home Beds to Meet Demand." *CNBC.com,* December 7.

McKinlay, John, and Lisa Marceau. 2008. "When There Is No Doctor: Reasons for the Disappearance of Primary Care Physicians in the US During the Early 21st Century." *Social Science and Medicine* 67:1481–91.

McKinstry, Brian. 1992. "Paternalism and the Doctor-Patient Relationship in General Practice." *British Journal of General Practice* 42:340–42.

McPherson, Chad Michael, and Michael Sauder. 2013. "Logics in Action: Managing Institutional Complexity in a Drug Court." *Administrative Science Quarterly* 58(2):165–96.

Mechanic, David. 1996. "Changing Medical Organization and the Erosion of Trust." *Milbank Quarterly* 74(2):171–89.

Mechanic, David. 2006. *The Truth About Health Care: Why Reform Is Not Working in America.* New Brunswick, NJ: Rutgers University Press.

Mechanic, David. 2008. "Rethinking Medical Professionalism: The Role of Information Technology and Practice Innovations." *Milbank Quarterly* 86(2):327–58.

Mechanic, David, and Donna D. McAlpine. 2010. "Sociology of Health Care Reform: Building on Research and Analysis to Improve Health Care." Supplement, *Journal of Health and Social Behavior* 51(S1):S147-59.

Mechanic, Robert, Kevin Coleman, and Allen Dobson. 1998. "Teaching Hospital Costs: Implications for Academic Missions in a Competitive Market." *JAMA* 280(11):1015–19.

Mello, Michelle M., David M. Studdert, Catherine M. DesRoches, Jordon Peugh, Kinga Zapert, Troyen A. Brennan, and William M. Sage. 2004. "Caring for Patients in a Malpractice Crisis: Physician Satisfaction and Quality of Care." *Health Affairs* 23(4):web exclusive. Retrieved March 24, 2022 (https://doi.org/10.1377/hlthaff.23.4.42).

Meyer, John, and Brian Rowan. 1977. "Institutionalized Organizations: Formal Structure as Myth and Ceremony." *American Journal of Sociology* 83(2):340–63

Meyer, John, W. Richard Scott, and David Strang. 1987. "Centralization, Fragmentation, and School District Complexity." *Administrative Science Quarterly* 32(2):186–201

Michalec, Barret. 2012. "The Pursuit of Medical Knowledge and the Potential Consequences of the Hidden Curriculum." *Health* 16(3):267–81.

Mickan, Sharon. 2005. "Evaluating the Effectiveness of Health Care Teams." *Australian Health Review: A Publication of the Australian Hospital Association* 29(2):211–7.

Millman, Marcia. 1977. *The Unkindest Cut: Life in the Backrooms of Medicine.* New York: William Morrow.

Mizrahi, Terry. 1986. *Getting Rid of Patients: Contradictions in the Socialization of Physicians.* New Brunswick, NJ: Rutgers University Press.

Morley, Chirstopher P., Carrie Roseamelia, Jordan A. Smith, and Ana L. Villarreal. 2013. "Decline of Medical Student Idealism in the First and Second Year of Medical School: A Survey of Pre-Clinical Medical Students at One Institution." *Medical Education Online* 18:1–10.

Mumford, Emily. 1970. *Interns: From Students to Physicians.* Cambridge, MA: Harvard University Press.

Mylotte, Joseph, Lucinda Kahler, and Carole McCann. 2001. "Community-Acquired Bacteremia at a Teaching Versus a Nonteaching Hospital: Impact of Acute Severity of Illness on 30-Day Mortality." *American Journal of Infection Control* 29(1):13–21.

Nancarrow, Susan A., and Alan M. Borthwick. 2005. "Dynamic professional boundaries in the health care workforce." *Sociology of Health and Illness* 27(7):897–919.

Newton, Bruce W., Laurie Barber, James Clardy, Elton Cleveland, and Patricia O'Sullivan. 2008. "Is There Hardening of the Heart During Medical School?" *Academic Medicine* 83(3):244–49.

Nyquist, Ann-Christine, Ralph Gonzales, John F. Steiner, and Merle A. Sande. 1998. "Antibiotics for Children with Upper Respiratory Infections." *Journal of the American Medical Association* 280:1401.

O'Connor, Nina, Paul Junker, Scott M. Appel, Robert Stetson, Jeffrey Rohrbach, and Salimah H. Meghani. 2018. "Palliative Care Consultation for Goals of Care and Future Acute Care Costs: A Propensity-Matched Study." *American Journal of Hospice and Palliative Medicine* 35(10):966–71.

O'Malley, Ann, and James D. Reschovsky. 2011. "Referral and Consultation Communication Between Primary Care and Specialist Physicians: Finding Common Ground." *JAMA Internal Medicine* 171(1):56–65.

Ocasio, William. 1998. "Towards an Attention-Based View of the Firm." Supplement, *Strategic Management Journal* 18(S1):187-206.

Ocloo, Josephine Enyonam. 2010. "Harmed Patients Gaining Voice: Challenging Dominant Perspectives in the Construction of Medical Harm and Patient Safety Reforms." *Social Science and Medicine* 71(3):510–16.

Organization for Economic Cooperation and Development (OECD). 2013. *Health at a Glance 2013: OECD Indicators.* Paris: OECD Publishing.

OECD. 2018. *Focus On: Spending on Health: Latest Trends.* Paris: OECD Publishing.

Oshima, Lee, Emily Emanuel, and Ezekiel J. Emanuel. 2013. "Shared Decision Making to Improve Care and Reduce Costs." *New England Journal of Medicine* 368(1):6–8.

Ozawa, Sachiko, and Pooja Sripad. 2013. "How Do You Measure Trust in the Health System? A Systematic Review of the Literature."" *Social Science and Medicine* 91(August):10–14.

Palmer, H. Carl Jr, et al. 2001. "The Effect of a Hospitalist Service with Nurse Discharge Planner on Patient Care in an Academic Teaching Hospital." *American Journal of Medicine* 111(8):627–32.

Parsons, Talcott. 1951. "Social Structure and Dynamic Process: The Case of Modern Medical Practice." In *The Social* System, 428–79. New York: Routledge.

Pearl, Robert. 2017. "Why Major Hospitals Are Losing Money By the Millions." *Forbes*. Retrieved March 20, 2019 (https://www.forbes.com/sites/robertpearl/2017/11/07/hospitals-losing-millions/?sh=3be876617b50).

Pirkle, Catherine M., Alexandre Dumont, and Maria-Victoria Zunzunegui. 2012. "Medical Recordkeeping, Essential But Overlooked Aspect of Quality of Care in Resource-Limited Settings." *International Journal of Quality Health Care* 24(6):546–67.

Polanyi, Karl. 1957[1944]. *The Great Transformation: The Political and Economic Origins of Our Time*. Boston: Beacon Press.

Popovic, J. R. 2001. "1999 National Hospital Discharge Survey: Annual Summary with Detailed Diagnosis and Procedure Data." *Vital and Health Statistics* 13(151):i–v. Retrieved March 24, 2022 (https://pubmed.ncbi.nlm.nih.gov/11594088/).

Quadagno, Jill. 2008. "Why the United States Has No National Health Insurance: Stakeholder Mobilization Against the Welfare State, 1945–1996." Supplement, *Journal of Health and Social Behavior* 45:25–44.

Quill, Timothy E., Robert M. Arnold, and Anthony L. Back. 2009. "Discussing Treatment Preferences with Patients Who Want 'Everything.'" *Annals of Internal Medicine* 151(5):345–49.

Pinsky, William W. 2000. "The Roles of Research in an Academic Medical Center." *Academic Affairs* 2(4): 201–2.

Rand, Cynthia M., Laura P. Shone, Christina Albertin, Peggy Auinger, Jonathan D. Klein, and Peter G. Szilagyi. 2007. "National Health Care Visit Patterns of Adolescents: Implications for Delivery of New Adolescent Vaccines." *Archives of Pediatrics & Adolescent Medicine* 161(3):252–59.

Rau, Jordan. 2012. "Medicare to Penalize 2,217 Hospitals for Excess Readmissions." *Kaiser Health News*, August 13.

Reed, Michael I. 1996. "Expert Power and Control in Late Modernity: An Empirical Review and Theoretical Synthesis." *Organization Studies* 17(4):573–97.

Reeder, Leo G. 1972. "The Patient-Client as a Consumer: Some Observations on the Changing Professional-Client Relationship." *Journal of Health and Social Behavior* 13(4):406–12.

Reich, Adam. 2014. *Selling Our Souls: The Commodification of Hospital Care in the United States*. Princeton, NJ: Princeton University Press.

Riska, Elianne. 2009. Gender and Medical Education. In *Handbook of the Sociology of Medical Education*, edited by C. Brosnan and B. S. Turner, 89–105. London: Routledge Taylor & Francis Group.

Roberts, Sam. 2012. "Nowhere to Go, Patients Linger in Hospitals, at a High Cost." *Herald Tribune*, January 2. Retrieved March 24, 2022 (https://www.heraldtribune.com/story/news/2012/01/02/nowhere-to-go-patients-linger/29072762007/).

Robinson, Glen O. 1986. "The Medical Malpractice Crisis of the 1970s: A Retrospective." *Law and Contemporary Problems* 49(2):5–35.

Romm, Fredric J., and Samuel M. Putnam. 1981. "The Validity of the Medical Record." *Medical Care* 19(3):310–15.

Rosoff, Stephen M., and Matthew C. Leone. 1991. "The Public Prestige of Medical Specialties: Overviews and Undercurrents." *Social Science and Medicine* 32(3):321–26.

Rossman, Gabriel. 2014. "Obfuscatory Relational Work and Disreputable Exchange." *Sociological Theory* 32(1):43–63.

Roter, Debra L., and Judith A. Hall. 2006. *Doctors Talking with Patients/Patients Talking with Doctors: Improving Communication in Medical Visits*. Westport, CT: Praeger.

Rothberg, Michael B., Joshua Class, Tara F. Bishop, Jennifer Friderici, Reva Kleppel, and Peter K. Lindenauer. 2014. "The Cost of Defensive Medicine on 3 Hospital Medicine Services." *JAMA Internal Medicine* 174(11):1867:68.

Salander, Pär, and Clare Moynihan. 2010. "Facilitating Patients' Hope Work Through Relationship: A Critique of the Discourse of Autonomy." In *Configuring Health Consumers: Health Work and the Imperative of Personal Responsibility*, edited by R. Harris, N. WA then, and S. Wyatt, 113–25. Houndmills, UK: Palgrave Macmillan.

Sanders, Tom, and Stephen Harrison. 2008. "Professional Legitimacy Claims in the Multidisciplinary Workplace: The Case of Heart Failure Care." *Sociology of Health and Illness* 30(2):289–308.

Sands, Roberta G., Judith Stafford, and Marleen McClelland. 1990. ""I beg to differ": Conflict in the Interdisciplinary Team." *Social Work in Health Care* 14(3):55-72.

Sanger-Katz, Margot. 2018. "Getting Sick Can Be Really Expensive, Even for the Insured." *New York Times*, March 21.

Scott, Tim, Russell Mannion, Martin Marshall, and Huw Davies. 2003. "Does Organisational Culture Influence Health Care Performance? A Review of the Evidence." *Journal of Health Services Research and Policy* 8(2):105–17.

Scott, W. Richard, Martin Ruef, Peter Mendel, and Carol A. Caronna. 2000. *Institutional Change and Health Care Organizations: From Professional Dominance to Managed Care.* Chicago: University of Chicago Press.

Serra, Helena. 2010. "Medical Technocracies in Liver Transplantation: Drawing Boundaries in Medical Practices." *Health* 14(2):162–77.

Shim, Janet K. 2010. "Cultural Health Capital: A Theoretical Approach to Understanding Health Care Interactions and the Dynamics of Unequal Treatment." *Journal of Health and Social Behavior* 51(1): 1–15.

Shortell, Stephen M., and Lawrence P. Casalino. 2008. "Health Care Reform Requires Accountable Care Systems. "*Journal of the American Medical Association* 300(1):95-7.

Shrank, William H., Teresa L. Rogstad, and Natasha Parekh. 2019. "Waste in the US Health Care System: Estimated Costs and Potential for Savings." *JAMA* 322(15):1501-09.

Shurtz, Ity. 2013. "The Impact of Medical Errors on Physician Behavior: Evidence from Malpractice Litigation." *Journal of Health Economics* 32(2):331–40.

Silbersweig, David R. 2016. "Harvard Medical Professor: The Nation's Teaching Hospitals Are under Threat." *Washington Post,* April 26.

Smith Jr., G. Randy, Jason M. Stein, and Mike C. Jones. 2012. "Acute Medicine in the United Kingdom: First-hand Perspectives on a Parallel Evolution of Inpatient Medical Care." *Journal of Hospital Medicine* 7(3):254-7.

Snoey, Eric. 2018. "'Just to Be Safe' Is Exactly the Wrong Reason to Get a Medical Test." *Los Angeles Times*, December 30. Retrieved March 19, 2019 (https://www.latimes.com/opinion/op-ed/la-oe-snoey-why-healthcare-is-plagued-by-overtesting-20181230-story.html).

Society of Hospital Medicine. 2011. *General Information about SHM.* Retrieved March 28, 2012 (http://www.hospitalmedicine.org/Content/NavigationMenu/AboutSHM/GeneralInformation/General_Information.htm).

Solheim, Karen, Beverly J. McElmurry, and Mi Ja Kim. 2007. "Multidisciplinary Teamwork in US Primary Health Care." *Social Science and Medicine* 65(3):622–34.

Sox, Harold C. 1999. "The Hospitalist Model: Perspectives of the Patient, the Internist, and Internal Medicine." *Annals of Internal Medicine* 130(4):368–72.

Starr, Paul. 1982. *The Social Transformation of American Medicine*. New York: Basic Books.

Stevens, Jennifer P., et al. 2015. "Variation in Inpatient Consultation among Older Adults in the United States." *Journal of General Internal Medicine* 30(7):992–99.

Stevenson, Fiona, Laura Hall, Maureen Seguin, Helen Atherton, Rebecca Barnes, Geraldine Leydon, Catherine Pope, Elizabeth Murray, and Sue Ziebland. 2018. "General Practitioner's Use of Online Resources During Medical Visits: Managing the Boundary Between Inside and Outside the Clinic." Supplement, *Sociology of Health and Illness* 41(S1): 65–81.

Street, Richard L. Jr., Gregory Makoul, Neeraj K. Arora, and Ronald M. Epstein. 2009. "How Does Communication Heal? Pathways Linking Clinician-Patient Communication to Health Outcomes." *Patient Education and Counseling* 74(3):295–301.

Studdert, David M., et al. 2000. "Negligent Care and Malpractice Claiming Behavior in Utah and Colorado." *Medical Care* 38(3):250–60.

Sutcliffe, Kathleen M., Elizabeth Lewton, and Marilynn M. Rosenthal. 2004. "Communication Failures: An Insidious Contributor to Medical Mishaps." *Academic Medicine* 79(2):186–94.

Szymczak, Julie E., and Charles L. Bosk. 2012. "Training for Efficiency: Work, Time, and Systems-Based Practice in Medical Residency." *Journal of Health and Social Behavior* 53(3):344–58.

Commonwealth Fund. 2015. *International Health Care System Profiles*. New York: Commonwealth Fund.

Terhune, Chad. 2017. "Putting A Lid On Waste: Needless Medical Tests Not Only Cost $200B—They Can Do Harm." *Kaiser Health News*, May 24. Retrieved March 16, 2022 (https://khn.org/news/putting-a-lid-on-waste-needless-medical-tests-not-only-cost-200b-they-can-do-harm/).

Thomas, Robert J. 1995. "Interviewing Important People in Big Companies." In *Studying Elites Using Qualitative Methods*, edited by R. Hertz and J. B. Imber, 3–17. Thousand Oaks, CA: Sage.

Thorlby, Ruth, and Sandeepa Arora. 2015. "The English Health Care System." *International Health Care System*. New York: Commonwealth Fund.

Thornton, Patricia H. 2004. *Markets from Culture: Institutional Logics and Organzational Decisions in Higher Education Publishing*. Palo Alto, CA: Stanford University Press.

Thornton, Patricia H., and William Ocasio. 1999. "Institutional Logics and the Historical Contingency of Power in Organizations: Executive Succession in the Higher Education Publishing Industry, 1958–1990." *American Journal of Sociology*, 105(3):801–43.

Thornton, Patricia H., and William Ocasio, eds. 2012. Institutional Logics. In *The Sage Handbook of Organizational Institutionalism*, 99–129. Thousand Oaks, CA: Sage.

Timmermans, Stefan. 1999. *Sudden Death and the Myth of CPR*. Philadelphia: Temple University Press.

Timmermans, Stefan, and Marc Berg. 2003. *The Gold Standard: The Challenge of Evidence-Based Medicine and Standardization in Health Care*. Philadelphia: Temple University Press.

Timmermans, Stefan, and Iddo Tavory. 2012. "Theory Construction in Qualitative Research: From Grounded Theory to Abductive Analysis." *Sociological Theory* 30(3):167–86.

Timmermans, Stefan. 2020. "The Engaged Patient: The Relevance of Patient-Physician Communication for Twenty-First-Century Health." *Journal of Health and Social Behavior* 61(3): 259–73.

Troyer, Lisa. 2004. "Democracy in a Bureaucracy: The Legitimacy Paradox of Teamwork in Organizations." in *Legitimacy Processes in Organizations, Research in the Sociology of Organizations*, edited by C. Johnson, 49–88. Bingley, UK: Emerald Group.

Underman, Kelly, and Laura E. Hirshfield. 2016. "Detached Concern? Emotional Socialization in Twenty-First Century Medical Education." *Social Science and Medicine* 160(July):94–101.

University of Michigan. n.d. "History of Michigan Medicine." Retrieved March 22, 2021 (https://www.uofmhealth.org/history).

Vento, Sandro, Francesca Cainelli, and Alfredo Vallone. 2018. "Defensive Medicine: It Is Time to Finally Slow Down an Epidemic." *World Journal of Clinical Cases* 6(11):406–09.

Voronov, Maxim, Dirk De Clercq, and C. R. Hinings. 2013. "Institutional Complexity and Logic Engagement: An Investigation of Ontario Fine Wine." *Human Relations* 66(12):1563–96.

Wachter, Robert M. 1999. "An Introduction to the Hospitalist Model." *Annals of Internal Medicine* 130(4 pt 2):338–42.

Wachter, Robert, and Lee Goldman. 2002. "The Hospitalist Movement 5 Years Later." *Journal of the American Medical Association* 287(4):487–94.

Waitzkin, Howard. 2000. "Changing Patient-Physician Relationships in the Changing Health-Policy Environment." In *Handbook of Medical Sociology*, vol. 5, edited by C. E. Bird, P. Conrad, and A. M. Fremont, 271–83. Upper Saddle River, NJ: Prentice Hall.

Wallack, Stanley S. 1992. "Managed Care: Practice, Pitfalls, and Potential." Annual Supplement, *Health Care Financing Review* 1991(March):27–34.

Wear, Delese, Julie M. Aultman, Joseph Varley, and Joseph Zarconi. 2006. "Making Fun of Patients: Medical Students' Perceptions and Use of Derogatory and Cynical Humor in Clinical Settings." *Academic Medicine* 81(5):454–62.

Weiss, Audrey J., and Anne Elixhauser. 2014. *Overview of Hospital Stays in the United States, 2012: Statistical Brief #108*. Rockville, MD: Agency for Health care Research and Quality.

Wells, R., Jinnett, K., Alexander, J., Lichtenstein, R., Liu, D., and Zazzali, J. L. (2006). Team Leadership and Patient Outcomes in US Psychiatric Treatment Settings. *Social Science and Medicine* 62(4, pt 2):1840–52.

Wennberg, John E., Elliott S. Fisher, David C. Gooodman, and Johnathan S. Skinner. 2008. *Tracking the Care of Patients with Severe Chronic Illness: The Dartmouth Atlas of Health Care 2008*. Lebanon, NH: Dartmouth Institute for Health Policy and Clinical Practice.

Wheeler, Daniel, Paul Marcus, Jenna Ngyuyen, Allison Kwong, Ali R. Khaki, Victoria Valencia, and Christopher Moriates. 2016. "Evaluation of a Resident-Led Project to Decrease Phlebotomy Rates in the Hospital: Think Twice, Stick Once." *JAMA Internal Medicine* 175(6):708-10.

Yin, Robert K. 2009. *Case Study Research: Design and Methods*, 4th ed. Thousand Oaks, CA: Sage.

Zelizer, Vivianna. 1979. *Morals and Markets: The Development of Life Insurance in the United States*. New York: Columbia University Press.

Zelizer, Vivanna. 2005. *The Purchase of Intimacy*. Princeton, NJ: Princeton University Press.

Zetka, James R. Jr. 2001. "Occupational Divisions of Labor and Their Technology Politics: The Case of Surgical Scopes and Gastrointestinal Medicine." *Social Forces* 79(4):1495–1520.

Zetka, James R. Jr. 2008. "The Making of the 'Women's Physician' in American Obstetrics and Gynecology: Re-Forging an Occupational Identity and a Division of Labor." *Journal of Health and Social Behavior* 49(3):335–51.

Zussman, Robert. 1992. *Intensive Care: Medical Ethics and the Medical Profession*. Chicago: University of Chicago Press.

Index

Abbott, Andrew, 10

abdominal pain, 41–42, 55, 62, 110

Abel, John Jacob, 12

academic medical centers: conflicting logics and, 4, 21–25, 28, 33, 37, 39; consultations and, 65, 71; economic issues and, 108, 119, 128; elite, 4, 11, 14, 17, 21, 61, 108, 129; intraprofessional dynamics at, 10; Reich on, 145n58; research and, 12, 21, 23–24, 37, 128, 139; training and, 13, 23, 119, 142; use of term, 139

accountability: conflicting logics and, 31; discharge and, 100; economic issues and, 122; malpractice, 21, 27–28, 59, 82, 99, 104, 110; medical records and, 44

Accreditation Council for Graduate Medical Education (ACGME), 38, 139

acute care, 8, 23, 26, 43, 89, 102, 142

administration: conflicting logics and, 24, 32, 35; cost-benefit analysis and, 13, 38, 43, 53–54, 76, 120, 129; dilemmas and, 1–2, 8; discharge and, 91; economic issues and, 24, 32, 35, 45, 60, 91, 107–8; increased complexity of, 7, 24, 32, 124; market logic and, 7–8, 11, 31; medical records and, 45, 60; research and, 132, 136

afternoon interdisciplinary rounds, 18, 133, 139

alcohol, 13

Allegheny Health, Education, and Research Foundation (AHERF), 30–31

almshouses, 22–23, 139, 146n5

Altomonte, Guillermina, 8–9, 43, 77, 119

Alzheimer's disease, 47

American Hospital Association, 52

American Medical Association (AMA), 27

CPSIA information can be obtained
at www.ICGtesting.com
Printed in the USA
JSHW061114260822
29738JS00001B/2